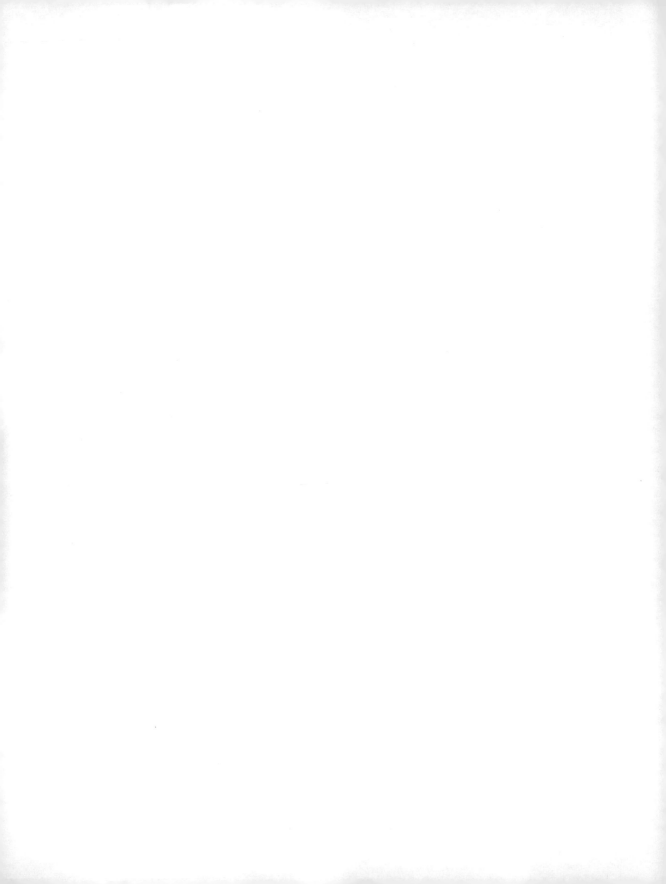

PRAISE FOR *Witness to Fitness*

"Donna is a trusted voice and highly respected leader who has helped millions become healthy from the inside out. Her energy and motivation are contagious and her heart to serve is pure."
　　　　　—Roland S. Martin, CNN analyst and TV One host of
　　　　　Washington Watch

"Donna Richardson Joyner is one of the most inspiring fitness gurus on the planet. In this groundbreaking new book, she will take you on a journey toward physical, emotional, and spiritual health. The time is now for you to become the best you can be."
　　　　　—Dr. Fabrizio Mancini, international bestselling author of
　　　　　The Power of Self-Healing

"If you can get people to believe that they are in charge of their own destiny, you enable them to transform their outcomes. Who is this book for? Anyone who wants to make a change."
　　　　　—Grant Hill, NBA forward for the Los Angeles Clippers

"*Witness to Fitness* will help you have victory in your health. Donna's wisdom, love, and encouragement will inspire you to achieve your goals in pursuit of good health, healing, and happiness."
　　　　　—Tracy and Alonzo Mourning, founders of the Mourning Family
　　　　　Foundation

"My friend Donna has traveled the world helping people to become healthier and live more meaningful lives. She is relentless when it comes to educating and empowering people to be faithful and fruitful when it comes to taking care of their bodies and souls."
　　　　　—Rev. Omarosa Manigault-Stallworth

"Donna has managed to integrate mind, body, and soul into a program that shows you how to combine faith, food, and fitness! Something we all need!"
　　　　　—Kirk and Tammy Franklin

WITNESS to FITNESS

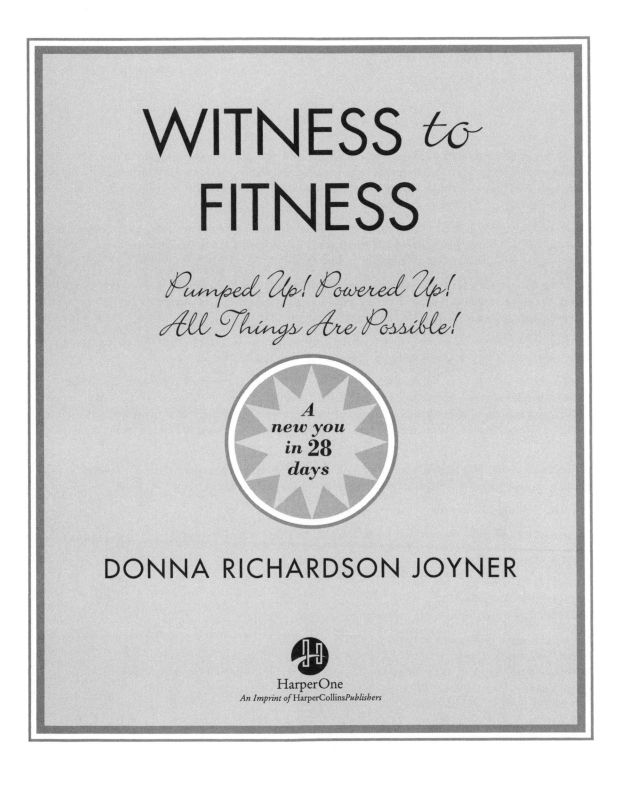

WITNESS *to* FITNESS

Pumped Up! Powered Up!
All Things Are Possible!

A
new you
in **28**
days

DONNA RICHARDSON JOYNER

HarperOne
An Imprint of HarperCollinsPublishers

HarperOne

Scripture quotations are taken from THE HOLY BIBLE, NEW INTERNATIONAL VERSION®, NIV®. Copyright © 1973, 1978, 1984, 2011 by Biblica, Inc.™ Used by permission. All rights reserved worldwide.

HarperCollins books may be purchased for educational, business, or sales promotional use. For information, please e-mail the Special Markets Department at SPsales@harpercollins.com.

HarperCollins website: http://www.harpercollins.com

HarperCollins®, 📖®, and HarperOne™ are trademarks of HarperCollins Publishers.

FIRST EDITION

Designed by Ralph Fowler
Photography by Rance Elgin
Vision tree illustration (page 29) by J. Lee Designs

Library of Congress Cataloging-in-Publication Data
Joyner, Donna Richardson.
Witness to fitness : pumped up! powered up! all things are possible! / Donna Richardson Joyner.
   p. cm.
  ISBN 978–0–06–211255–2
  1. Exercise. 2. Physical fitness. 3. Nutrition. 4. Mind and body. 5. Exercise for women. I. Title.
  RA781.J74 2013
  613.7'1—dc23   2012028379

13 14 15 16 17 RRD(H) 10 9 8 7 6 5 4 3 2 1

This book is dedicated to my beloved grandmother

Ruth Naomi Cash

CONTENTS

FOREWORD

I have spent my life helping individuals become as healthy as possible in every dimension of their lives: spiritually, emotionally, psychologically, and physically. Having warred with my own weight and fought my way back to fitness after numerous injuries and subsequent surgeries, I know personally the multitudinous benefits of a healthy body. As the pastor of the Potter's House and our more than 30,000 members, I have witnessed too many people succumb to illness before fulfilling their God-given potential.

And it's not an isolated problem. According to Dr. Regina Benjamin, the U.S. surgeon general, "Two-thirds of Americans are overweight or obese." All of us battle with eating a well-balanced, nutritious diet and getting enough proper exercise to stay healthy and fit. Two out of three of us are losing this battle right now. You may be at risk for diabetes or heart disease. You may be increasing your risk of cancer by your lifestyle habits. You may need to drop some pounds to increase your energy level and enjoyment of life.

But no one changes until they're sick and tired of being sick and tired. You must be willing to diagnose your denial and make new choices that are integrated with all the other areas of your life. You cannot conquer what you're not committed to carrying forward. You cannot win at what you're not willing to welcome. God gave you a body in his image and wants you to care for it as his temple. I'm convinced it's a form of worship to notice, nourish, and nurture the temple with which he's blessed you.

I've never seen an individual who shares this belief with more conviction than Donna Richardson Joyner. As her pastor, I've experienced her passion for merging faith and fitness and witnessed her dedication to wellness on every level. Her comprehensive program will inspire you to live a more productive, powerful, and purposeful life. In these pages you will discover her selfless and relentless desire to energize you to new levels of spiritual and physical vitality.

Don't wait until you've lost your health to realize just how important it is. Too often we forget to be grateful for feeling good until we're feeling bad. Donna's blend of motivation, inspiration, and perspiration will help you sow an eternal investment even as you reap the healthiest of returns right now. Isn't it time for you to make the most of what you've been given? Isn't it time to give yourself the gift of a healthy mind, body, and soul? If you're ready to experience a fresh start and a whole new level of wholeness, then turn the page, and as Donna says, "Let's get pumped up, powered up, and prayed up!"

—Bishop T. D. Jakes

WITNESS *to* FITNESS

INTRODUCTION

I haven't walked in your shoes and you haven't in mine. But I'm sure we have experienced some of the same struggles, setbacks, and frustrations in life. I'm here to share with you love, knowledge, and experience to help you transform your health and your life. I've learned to decrease self-interest and increase God's interest so that I can better serve, inspire, and elevate you. The focus of this journey is not about where you have been but about where you are going. You can't change your past health but you can change your future well-being.

I have traveled from city to city, country to country, helping people live healthier and more purposeful lives. I have worked with the rich, the poor, the overweight, the undernourished, the willing, the reluctant, the hopeful, and the hopeless. My greatest challenge was not overseas; it was my family, my community, and my church. I was sick and tired of being sick and tired of seeing loved ones:

- suffer from preventable illnesses,
- go to heaven way too soon,
- know better but not do better, and
- be prisoners of their own health.

It's time for change, and you have the power to make change happen. Change does not occur on the outside until it has manifested on the inside. Why wait for bad health to come knocking at your door when you can do something now and experience the joy of good health? Your health is the power line of your life, so take steps to recharge and renew.

Are you ready to walk in the newness in your health and in your life? Act now, because tomorrow is not promised to you. Do it while you can, because there comes a time when you can't. First, you have to change your thinking and get a new attitude. Second, strengthen your spirit and see God's light. Walk by faith and not by sight. And last, move and eat to win and be victorious in managing your health. My goal is to help you get the results you are destined for, live life more abundantly, and create lasting change for generations to come.

Pumped up! Powered up! All things are possible!
Be a witness to fitness!
—Donna

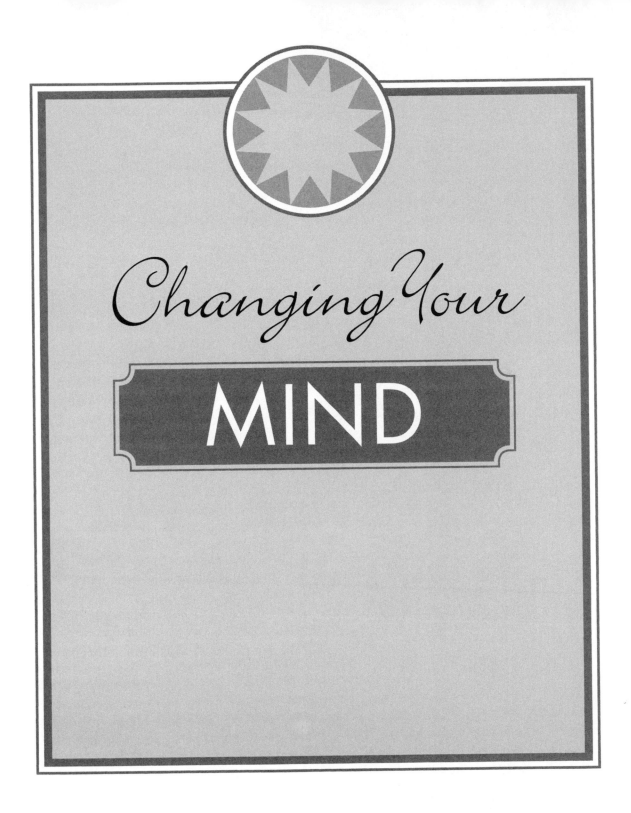

Changing Your

MIND

Transforming Your Mind-Set

'Ve had an It's Possible list for several years now to help me organize, prioritize, and visualize my dreams. It's sort of my version of the standard bucket list, only less depressing, and something more than a wish list, because that isn't definitive enough for me. One of the items on my It's Possible list was to climb Mount Kilimanjaro, the tallest freestanding mountain in the world at 19,340 feet. So you can imagine how excited I was when an opportunity presented itself. I trained hard for two solid months, preparing myself for the difficult climb, and then the call came—the deal was off. I was very disappointed that my It's Possible climb was no longer possible.

Several months had passed since that disappointing news, and my It's Possible list still had climbing Mount Kilimanjaro on it. As I stared at my list, I thought, "Why am I depending on someone else to make this happen when I can do it myself?" This wasn't beyond my reach, so I decided to go for it.

That November, during my forty-eighth birthday party, I announced that I was going to climb Mount Kilimanjaro as a birthday goal and gift to give back. I asked if anyone wanted to join me on the journey. Two of my dear friends, Rockin' Raquel and Super Shannay, said they wanted to go, and "Ready Rance" Greer, a renowned photographer and videographer, would document the feat. So the training began again.

By the time we left for Tanzania, I was ready mentally, physically, emotionally, and spiritually. The preparation was tough, but the process of getting to the mountaintop proved the most difficult. When I thought I couldn't take another step, I would sing the lyrics to that James Cleveland song "I Don't Believe He Brought Me This Far to Leave Me." I sang it loud and off-key most of the time, but I was definitely making a joyful noise unto the Lord.

SWEET TWEET

Anything can happen when U believe. Don't fret or let go before U achieve.

Move every mountain out of your way. God is able 2 answer today!

Courage, perseverance, and faith took me up and then down that mountain. No matter how painful and labor intensive, I kept going. I dug deep into my belly and grabbed hold of the inner strength I needed to push ahead. Although the climb tested the very fabric of my being, I was victorious in accomplishing my goal. I climbed to the top of that majestic mountain and declared, "With God all things are possible!" I could now check off one big item from my It's Possible list.

We not only climbed the mountain, we also did missionary work and visited area orphanages, giving them food, school supplies, uniforms, soccer balls, and more importantly love. We spoke to them about having courage, faith, and perseverance. It was an unforgettable, life-changing experience, and it all began with one step in the right direction. I put into action a dream on my It's Possible list, and God was with me every step of that amazing experience.

At the beginning of this journey, I thought it would be a personal milestone, but I soon realized it was much bigger than me, my milestones, and my It's Possible list. I realize now that I climbed that mountain for you. I climbed that mountain so I could say to you, "There is no mountain too big for our God. No matter what obstacle you're facing today, you can conquer it and be victorious."

Decide and Conquer

You probably wouldn't have picked up this book if you weren't battling health issues, struggling to lose weight, or desperately trying to get fit. Well, I have good news—you made the right decision, because the answers you need to transform your health and your life are here in this book. How do I know? Because I am living proof that when your health is important to you, you can refresh, re-store, and rejuvenate your being and live your life to the fullest.

It all starts with a decision to act on your dreams. See, if I hadn't made the decision to go after my dream of climbing the tallest mountain in the world, that item would still be on my It's Possible list, and I'd be another year older, still dreaming about it but never achieving it. Or what if I had planned the whole trip, climbed halfway up the mountain, and announced, "This is just too difficult. I think I'll go back home"? I would've gone home defeated, wondering if I could've made it up that mountain if I'd only pushed a little harder.

How about you? How many times have you started a diet on Monday, but by Wednesday given up and devoured a bag of cookies? Or joined a gym on January 1, gone five times that first week, but not been back since? Listen, we've all been there. We've all made that initial decision to improve our health and then become overwhelmed and frustrated carrying out our goals. But this time is different, because I'm going to give you the tools to conquer this once and for all. We are going to decide and conquer—together.

I'm not saying this will be an easy journey. My climb up Mount Kilimanjaro wasn't easy, but it was so fulfilling in the end. Your journey will be rewarding too, but you have to decide right now that you want to transform your health and your life. And you have to decide that you're willing to do whatever it takes to make those dreams come to fruition.

Change, Renew, and Do

When people ask me, "What is the most important thing you can do to become fit and lose weight?" I think they are surprised by my answer. I don't tell them about a magic pill or a ridiculous diet. I simply say, "You have to change your mind-set—period." If you change your thinking, your actions will change, because your thoughts govern your actions. Proverbs 23:7 says it like this: "For as he thinks in his heart, so is he." So what are you? A believer, not a doubter. An overcomer, not an underachiever. The head, not the tail. You're above, not beneath. A winner, not a loser. You're the headlight, not the taillight.

Say this out loud: "If change is to be, it's up to me." We have to change the "I can't do" mentality to the "I can do all things" mentality. Think of it as changing the stations on your radio. When the song "Doom, Despair, and Agony on Me" comes on, hit the scan button until you find a station playing "New Attitude" and stay there. Remember that song by Patti LaBelle? She said, "I'm feeling good from my head to my shoes . . . I've tidied up my point of view, I've got a new attitude." You're singing along right now, aren't you? Good! I want you to sing along, because I want that new-attitude thinking to become rooted in your heart.

It's a fact: if you change your thinking, you'll change where you're going. The "I can'ts" and "I don'ts" never moved anyone forward. It's time to get rid of that negative self-talk and self-loathing. Your past health is behind you, and your new health is in front of you. When you move forward, you can't think like you used to, because it will limit your ability to achieve what's in front of you. Participate in the production of becoming a better you.

Love Yourself Better Than That

Singer Shirley Murdock wrote a song called "I Love Me Better Than That," and I find myself singing her powerful lyrics all the time. I think this should be our anthem as we work out this mind-spirit-body transformation. If we don't love ourselves,

TRANSFORMATION *Tidbits*

- No matter what obstacle you're facing today, you can conquer it and be victorious.

- You have to value your health in order to make a commitment with your time, your energy, and your money.

- If you change your thinking, you'll change where you're going.

- You have to want to change more than you want to stay the same.

- Make a choice, not an excuse!

- Once you forgive, you abandon contaminated space.

we can't love anybody else, and we can't fulfill our purpose here on this earth. Maybe you didn't grow up in a loving home where your parents affirmed you daily. Maybe your home life isn't filled with lots of love and encouragement. Stop looking for approval from others. Go to your Heavenly Father for approval. Guess what? He's already given you his ultimate stamp of approval; you just have to receive it.

Often people don't approve of themselves because they are too busy comparing themselves to others. They get caught up in wanting to look like Victoria's Secret models and airbrushed photos of celebrities in magazines, but here's what I tell all who fall into that comparison trap: "Just do you!" Stop trying to be somebody else, and be who the Creator made you to be! It's too exhausting trying to be somebody else. Love yourself for who you are, right where you are, on the way to where you're going.

Do you love yourself enough to invest your time, energy, prayer, power, and heart into this process?

If not, we have some work to do on your inside before your miracle can manifest on the outside. Self-love and stinkin' thinkin' cannot coexist in your mind. It's time to start loving yourself, get rid of destructive thoughts, and shake loose all the excuses you've been using for years. That's what one of my clients, Dawn, had to do.

I first met Dawn while I was doing an appearance at an event in Orlando, Florida. She waited in a long line, and when she finally had my attention, she let me know that she wanted more than a signed fitness video. She was crying out for help, so I asked her to wait until the signing was over so I could meet with her one-on-one.

Dawn's story was heartbreaking, but after hearing it, I knew that she could overcome her struggle and eventually taste the sweetness of success. She had let her weight climb to more than 400 pounds, and she wanted to find out how to get her life back—not just for herself, but also for her young son. Through tears, she shared how she could no longer fly to see her relatives in other states because she couldn't fit into one airplane seat and couldn't afford to buy two tickets to accommodate her size. She had to ask total strangers to ride the roller coasters and other amusement-park rides with her son because she was too big to fit in the seats. She said she was working on getting a master's degree, but she was thinking of dropping out because she couldn't fit into any of the chairs in the classrooms. But the final heartbreak, the moment of reckoning, had come when she was enrolling her son in kindergarten. As she sat with her son's teacher, Dawn had felt the chair start to buckle beneath her weight. She prayed, "God, if you'll let me get through this without embarrassing myself or my son, I'll do better." She made it through the kindergarten enrollment, and then made her way to my video signing.

I told her what I'm telling you now: You have to change your mind-set and start moving toward better health for you! You didn't get to this weight overnight; so don't expect to lose the weight overnight. Lastly, you have to be sick and tired of being sick and tired of where you are, and have the desire to do something different. Don't be a prisoner of your own health; take charge. Don't be bound. Be free! Be loosed! Let's touch and agree.

More than 240 pounds later, Dawn has achieved her goal weight. She finished a half marathon with me last year; she attained her master's degree in education; and she's a teacher, helping others improve their lives. Let me be real: if Dawn can do it, you can do it. When I start my speaking engagements, I get people fired up by saying, "Get powered up, pumped up, and prayed up!" Get powered up for a total transformation! Get pumped up to be healthy and whole! Get prayed up for a better way of life! In the book of James it says faith without works is dead, so we have to work it! My grandmother always said it this way: "If you take one step, the good Lord will take two." James Brown's interpretation of that same message is "Get up offa that thing." And First Lady Michelle Obama says, "Let's move!" I echo all of those mantras—it's time to move it!

No More Excuses

About twenty years ago I was walking down the street with my fitness mentor, Charles, and this woman looked me up and down and said, "Girl, you stole my body. I was supposed to have your body!" Before I could respond to her, Charles said, "No, I don't think so. If you continue to wolf down those chili cheese fries, that hot dog, and that Big Gulp, there will be two of you instead of one." It was the truth spoken in love, and that woman ended up coming to our classes and developing her best body. She discovered that her healthy body had been there all along; she just had to work to uncover it. So do you!

As a fitness guru, I've heard every excuse imaginable, and I'm not having any of them! The woman with the chili cheese fries and hot dog had to get rid of her excuses for not eating healthy and never finding the time for fitness, and so do you, because excuses are the main barriers to your transformation. You will never make progress if you hold on to your reasons for not eating right or being active. I like to say it this way: you've made an excuse; now make a choice.

The most common excuse I hear from people is not having enough time to exercise. Time is really a matter of priorities. If you need or value something, you will invest your time, money, and energy in it. Do you need or value your health? If so, you'll make it a priority.

People come to my seminars with nice-looking hair and perfect nails, and I know they've spent some quality time in a salon getting groomed, but they stand there and tell me they don't have time to fit in fitness. These same people can tell you the story line of several different TV dramas they watch faithfully each week, but they can't find time to work out. I'm not buying it, I'm not hearing it, and I'm definitely not receiving it.

What if your doctor sat you down and asked, "Would you rather exercise one hour of every day or be dead every hour of every day?" How would you respond? Exercising an hour every day wouldn't seem so bad after all, would it? Well, that's what I'm saying to you—you have to make time for movement. You can multitask—watch your favorite TV dramas while on the treadmill—but just make time to move! If your health matters to you, and I think it does or you wouldn't have picked up this book, then you must invest your time, energy, and money in taking care of your-

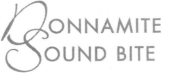

BONNAMITE SOUND BITE

You may be knocked down, but you're not out. Get off your butt, and say with a shout, "I'll be victorious—there ain't no doubt!"

self. Schedule working out and eating healthy like you would a doctor, business, or hair appointment. Speaking for myself, I rarely miss a hair appointment. Make a choice, not an excuse!

Here are three other common excuses I hear:

I'M TOO FAT TO EXERCISE. No matter what shape or size you are, you can reap the benefits of a healthy lifestyle. I'm not asking you to run a marathon your first day out; I'm simply asking you to start doing some physical activity for ten to twenty minutes each day. It's all about building up gradually. Water aerobics is a good option to start with, since it puts less stress on your joints and has a low impact on your body. If you combine being physically active with better nutrition, the weight will start to fall off and you will feel so much better. Take little steps that will lead to big accomplishments. Make a choice, not an excuse!

I'M TOO OLD TO EXERCISE. If you can move, you're not too old (or too heavy) to groove. You can be active at any age, just make sure you start with activities that are low impact and less stressful, like chair aerobics, walking, swimming, or stretching. People ask me, "Donna, what's the best exercise?" And I say, "The one you do." Regardless of your age, your health is a necessity. Without it you can't continue to rise, shine, and succeed in your life's journey. We don't want to just grow old and retire; we want to grow old and refire! Don't you want to be able to walk up a flight of steps and not be winded, or dance at a party and not run out of steam? Don't you want to be a role model and be active with your kids, or play with your grandkids? Then you have to move! I'll tell you, when I reached age fifty I increased my commitment to eating healthier and added extra workouts to my weekly routine because my metabolism has slowed down. I remember looking in the mirror one day and noticing how things had changed; it was nothing nice. I said to myself, this is not acceptable. I just had to become more committed and disciplined, like I tell others. Make a choice, not an excuse!

IT'S TOO EXPENSIVE TO WORK OUT. Negative! You have to change your mind-set about how you invest in your health. Your health is a necessity, not a luxury. We spend money on items like iPhones, BlackBerrys, iPads, purses, shoes, big screen TVs, new cars, etc., because we obviously value these items. Now I'm asking you to spend money on your health. Imagine what the return will be. Plus, the cost of not investing in your health will be far greater than the minimum cost to improve your health. Just a reminder: walking, dancing, jogging, and playing outside are free. For a nominal cost you can purchase a jump rope, dumbbells, fitness DVDs, and resistance bands, to name a few. You have to value your health enough to invest in it and get a good return. Make a choice, not an excuse!

Don't Let Your Guard Down

Say this out loud: "God can't bless what I don't do." The bottom line is, you have to want to change more than you want to stay the same. It's important that you don't become too comfortable where you are; if you do, you'll end up staying there. Trust me—it is dangerous to do nothing. I know because I've been in that do-nothing land before. There was a time in my life when I was simply existing and allowing my situation to control me. I had given up my inner power. I felt so weak that I didn't have the strength to fight my way back to the land of moving forward, so I simply settled there and became complacent. That's a dangerous place to dwell, because you tend to let your guard down.

I saw this same thing play out when I watched a big fight between Floyd "Money" Mayweather and Victor Ortiz. At one point in the fight, the boxers had to be separated because Ortiz illegally headbutted Mayweather. After Ortiz apologized and hugged Mayweather, the referee motioned for the

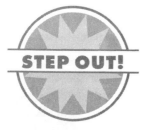

Habakkuk 2:2 says to "write the vision and make it plain on tablets, that he may run who reads it." That's what I want you to do. Remember my It's Possible list? I want you to make your own It's Possible list and get excited about where you're going. Make your list and check it twice. Don't delay. Start today and pray.

fight to begin again. Ortiz, however, decided to go in for one last apology, and in the process, he let his guard down. Mayweather took full advantage of Ortiz's mistake and clocked him with his trademark left hook, followed by a hard right, sending Ortiz plummeting to the floor. Ortiz was down for the count, all because he had let his guard down.

You see, when you're living on Complacency Street in Do-Nothing County, you let your guard down just long enough to get punched and maybe even knocked out by circumstances you hadn't foreseen. But grab hold of your inner strength and fight back. You're not knocked out! Get up, and fight with faith! Fight to win! This is where negative self-talk has to be silenced. Say to yourself, "I love me, and no matter what, I am pushing through!" When you let negative self-talk creep into your life, you're actually cursing yourself. What comes out of your mouth should bless you, not curse you. Your words should bring life, not death. Joel Osteen, pastor of Lakewood Church, recently said something small but compelling. He began his sermon with two simple words—*I am*. Then he said, "You choose what follows *I am*." That's good, isn't it? Psalm 139:14 says, "I am fearfully and wonderfully made." That's a good way to finish that sentence. Even if you can't think of anything else positive to say after *I am*, you can declare, "I am fearfully and wonderfully made."

What you say about yourself matters. In the movie *The Help*, Aibileen, the feisty maid, tells the young girl she cares for to repeat these words every day: "I is kind. I is smart. I is important." Grammatically correct or not, those are powerful words to say to yourself. Every morning when I wake up and am blessed with another day of my life, I say out loud, "Rise, shine, and succeed!" Now, there are days when that light is a little dim and success seems miles away, but on those days, I push and press through to glory. No matter what my cir-

cumstances, no matter how I feel, and no matter what happened yesterday, I give thanks and I keep charging ahead. I stay upbeat and focus on positive thoughts, so that I don't plant negative seeds that bring forth a negative harvest.

Unfortunately, that's what happened to a well-known major-league baseball pitcher named José Lima. Most baseball fans remember José Lima. He gained a reputation for greatness as a starting pitcher for the Houston Astros in the late 1990s. This talented pitcher learned about the power of words the hard way. When the Astros built their new stadium, the fence in left field was quite a bit closer than it had been in the Astrodome. In fact, Minute Maid Park has one of the shortest distances from home plate to the left-field fence of any baseball park in the entire country. It is considered one of the top ten environments for hitters, which is bad news for pitchers.

When José Lima stood on the pitcher's mound and noticed the close proximity of the left-field fence, he said, "I'll never be able to pitch in here." And do you know that he had one of the worst seasons of his career? He went from being a twenty-game winner to a sixteen-game loser in back-to-back seasons. See, José Lima allowed those negative thoughts to defeat him—first in his mind, then when he spoke them out of his mouth. So release those negative thoughts and silence that negative self-talk. Replace them with positive thinking, positive words, and positive actions.

Forgive and Live

Sometimes it's not your negative self-talk that stops you from succeeding; it's the negative words of those around you. You may be surrounded by people who are not championing you and celebrating you; instead, they may be poisoning you and discouraging you. I want you to think about the people in your life. Picture them as elevator buttons. Which ones are they? Are they the UP button, lifting you up with encouragement and kind words? Or are they the DOWN button, speaking negatively about your dreams and making fun of your progress? If they take you down, they don't need to be around. Fill your space, your home, and your work with people who build you up.

I realize you don't necessarily get to choose your coworkers—or your family, for that matter. If those people are negative forces in your life and you can't walk away from them, you're going to have to shield yourself from their hurtful remarks and counteract their words with God's word. When your coworker says, "I see that you've lost some weight. Well, don't go buy a new wardrobe yet because you'll probably just gain back that weight. Most people do, and they usually put on more weight than they lost," shake it off. That coworker is definitely a DOWN button, but you don't have to take that ride down. When any negative thoughts enter your mind, tell yourself, "Access denied." Meditate on positive thoughts and take positive actions. Tell yourself, "I'm letting go of my pain so I can move forward to healing, hope, peace, and joy."

You may have been in some bad relationships where people said hurtful things to you, and you replay their words over and over again. Their destructive words have become a blessing blocker in your life, because they have stopped you from moving forward. Listen, it doesn't matter who

mistreated you; use it as fuel to strengthen your spirit and breathe hope into your heart. It's time to forgive and live.

Once you forgive, you abandon that contaminated space and move into a space of freedom. Forgiving those people frees you from their words. It's time to rise above the pain and take back your power. See, when you forgive others, you take away their power to hurt you. I know that's easier said than done, but you have to forgive them if you want to move forward and continue your mission. Holding on to grudges and past offenses leads to self-doubt and low self-esteem, which leaves you paralyzed and powerless. Eventually, you'll become bitter and live in a sort of mental lockdown, imprisoned by the past you've held on to for too long. No more! Say, "No more!" Ask God to help you forgive those people. Let his love heal and make you whole. Forgive by faith, and freedom will come.

The Creator put you on this earth for a purpose. You can't accomplish that purpose if you're unhealthy, and you can't become totally whole mentally, physically, or spiritually until you let go through forgiveness. Turn your hurting into healing. Don't stay lame; shake off the blame! Give birth to your dreams and power to your purpose. Meditate on Isaiah 54:17: "No weapon formed against you shall prosper, and every tongue which rises against you in judgment you shall condemn." Rise up and say, "I'm a fighter, not a quitter!" Do it now and allow your faith to propel you forward. That's a huge step toward wellness and living life fully.

Stronger Than Any Stronghold

The road to total wellness is not always a smooth one. Sometimes you will experience strongholds in your life that have kept you from being committed to your health. I meet people who claim they are ready to embrace change, yet they are stalled. If you are consumed with your past, how do you stretch toward your future? I tell them, "Take authority over those strongholds. Don't let them take authority over you!"

What is a spiritual stronghold? I like evangelist Edgardo Silvoso's definition best: "A spiritual stronghold is a mind-set impregnated with hopelessness that causes us to accept as unchangeable situations that we know are contrary to the will of God." Basically, a stronghold is anything in your life that you've allowed to remain, even though you know it is keeping you from accomplishing the goals that are in your heart.

What are your strongholds? Do you have anything keeping you from achieving your health goals? I've met people around the world who are improving their lives through health and wellness, and I've noticed there are four common strongholds that keep them from moving forward: fear, generational curses, complacency, and hopeless-

ness. I want to face each of these strongholds head-on and give you the tools to overcome each one.

FEAR: People tell me all the time, "Donna, I have tried every gadget, diet, and pill on the market, and I am still overweight and out of shape." I can see the fear in their eyes—fear of failing at yet another attempt at losing weight and getting fit. My response? "I don't doubt that you've tried everything and the outcome wasn't successful. My program has God at the center, and it's important for you to have a health covenant with him. It's about living and practicing the word of good health and well-being."

Not only does the fear of failure keep people from stepping out in faith. The fear of success

---

SWEET TWEET

When U are 2 heavy 2 pick up the broken pieces, in total praise he increases.

With blinded eyes, take your faith walk. Move, don't U talk!

can be just as crippling. There's a scene in a baseball movie called *Summer Catch*, starring Freddie Prinze Jr. and Jessica Biel, that really speaks to me. Freddie plays a pitcher with a huge chip on his shoulder—very talented but always sabotaging his success because of his fear. He tries to convince himself that he'll be content mowing yards the rest of his life, but Jessica knows he can do so much more. The night before the biggest game of his life, where all the major-league scouts will be scrutinizing him, she looks him straight in the eyes and says, "Let yourself be great tomorrow." In other words, let your greatness shine through and stop allowing your fears to hinder your success. Make a paradigm shift in your mind-set, and turn your fear into your power. Don't let the stronghold of fear keep you bound. Don't let the fear of failure keep you from trying. Billie Jean King once said, "Failure is feedback on the road to success." Don't let the fear of success keep you from stepping out in faith.

This is a new day, and I have a new way! Follow me because we're headed for victory! Don't let

TRANSFORMATION *Tidbits*

- You can't achieve your purpose if you're unhealthy and sitting on the sidelines of life.

- Be relentless and radical in your pursuit of good health.

- A stronghold is anything in your life that you've allowed to remain, even though you know it is keeping you from accomplishing the goals in your heart.

- With hope, you won't just survive; you'll thrive!

- You are stronger than any stronghold!

fear cripple you anymore. Fear is the opposite of faith, and it takes faith to overcome fear. Remember, 2 Timothy 1:7 tells us that we weren't given a spirit of fear but of power, love, and a sound mind. Therefore, if the spirit of fear wasn't given to us, we don't want it. If you trust in God for everything else in your life, why not trust in him for your health?

GENERATIONAL STRONGHOLDS: I was always a very active child. I was involved in sports and recreational activities, and I remember looking at some of my relatives who were overweight and saying to my mother, "Am I going to be overweight too?" My mom responded, "Honey, you just keep staying active and you're going to be fine." If illnesses such as obesity, diabetes, and others are rampant in your family, take action and bring about change. Don't let generational health strongholds rob you of your life. Fight them every step of the way! Be proactive about your health.

Go to a doctor on a regular basis and know what your health status is. Begin eating to live, not living to eat. Consume foods that will nourish your body, not sabotage your health. We'll talk in detail about what to eat in chapter 7, but you have to decide that you're going to eat healthier. Set an example for your children: if you're telling your children they can't have any sugar, but you're eating half a dozen donuts on your way home from work, you're not fooling anybody, including your children.

Take control over those generational strongholds—the diseases that plague your family tree and the unhealthy habits you learned from family members. Don't use those things as an excuse to remain the same. Generational strongholds are not accepted. Put a stamp on them that says NOT APPROVED! Listen, you have to be accountable for your health, and you can't achieve your purpose if you are unhealthy and sitting on the sidelines of life. So get radical and be relentless in your pursuit

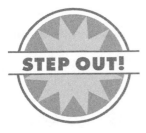

STEP OUT! On a blank piece of paper, write the name of your stronghold. Now, as an active step in the right direction, take that piece of paper, crumple it up, and throw it into the trash. As you're doing this very deliberate act, envision yourself being set free from that stronghold.

of good health. If you stay lukewarm, nothing will change. Get fired up! Your actions will break any generational strongholds. No longer should you be a prisoner of your own health. Be loosed! Be free! It's time to take a step toward reviving your soul, renewing your spirit, and restoring your body.

COMPLACENCY: Pastor A. R. Bernard of the Christian Cultural Center in Brooklyn, New York, says, "My alarm clock wakes me up, but my goals get me out of bed." I love that! We all need goals to get us out of bed each day and keep us motivated. If you're living in that warm, comfy bed of life, never stepping out to go after your dreams, that's a stronghold of complacency. Maybe you've convinced yourself that those last 15 to 30 pounds are okay; I mean, you look better than most people your age. Or maybe you've settled into a routine that doesn't involve any physical activity, but you justify your complacency because you take the stairs once in a while. Ask yourself whether your thoughts are hindering you or empowering you.

Unfortunately, in our society we are prone to less movement. Or I should call it like it is: laziness. We name furniture after our slothful ways: La-Z-Boy and recliner. I think we should have an action chair that looks like other nice furniture, but if you sit in it too long, the chair pokes you, music starts to play, and you get your butt up and move. You may think this sounds crazy, but I will do whatever is in my power to get America and the world up and moving.

Don't let laziness set up camp in your life! Command lazybones out! Think *move*! And let go of complacency and laziness. When you feel like you can't move forward, complacency and laziness will lead you to feeling stuck or trapped. It's the worst attack on your mind, but you can't let it take authority. Keep moving forward, and stop justifying why you can't achieve your goals. It's tempting to give yourself a license to stay where you are, but there's a danger in remaining in neutral. It's sort of like treading water. Sure, you'll stay in the same place for a while, but eventually you need to get motivated and swim to shore, or you'll go under. You're going over, not under! You're an overcomer, right? It's time to step out of your comfort zone and go after your dreams! Don't keep going back to an old comfortable space. I want you to go to a space of newness and wholeness, so you can live exceedingly, abundantly, and beyond all you could ever imagine.

HOPELESSNESS: Hopelessness is the despair you feel when you have abandoned the hope of success. Of all the strongholds I encounter, hopelessness is the most debilitating, because without hope, a person becomes totally paralyzed. Sometimes when I am coaching, I can tangibly feel hopelessness emanating from a person. I can sense a broken spirit, and I know that before that person can receive anything, I am going to have to deal with the stronghold of hopelessness.

Proverbs 13:12 says, "Hope deferred makes the heart sick." You see, without hope you have no faith, you have no vision, and you have no drive to accomplish your goals. Plus, you have no joy, because hope and joy are close friends. In fact, you can't have joy without hope, which means you can't have strength either, because Nehemiah 8:10 tells us that the joy of the Lord is our strength. Hopelessness will keep you in a depressed state so long that your faith will atrophy, and you'll eventually be too weak to strive for more. That's why you can't allow yesterday's sorrow to follow you into tomorrow.

I understand that you may have encountered challenges and disappointments in life, but don't allow those emotions to dictate your future. When I have experienced tough times in my life, despair and doom could not become my friends. No matter how difficult the situation was, I would not allow my mind to be filled with defeat. I did everything within my power to focus and take action for a positive outcome. And when something was beyond my reach, I asked God to step in. Your faith in him turns hopelessness to hopefulness, negative to positive, and impossible to possible. Think of hope as your trump card. Whenever you are facing an obstacle, remember God is bigger. He reigns!

Breaking-Free Strategies

Whether you're struggling with generational strongholds or the strongholds of fear, complacency, or hopelessness, these strategies will help you break free:

1. DEFINE: Start by defining the problem. Write it down. Admit your present condition instead of staying in denial mode. Accept responsibility for where you are and, most important, be truthful.

2. CREATE: Create an action plan and work the plan. You have to be a worker bee.

> ### BONNAMITE SOUND BITE
>
> No more strongholds in my life. I'm leaving those behind. I'm stepping out in faith today. Sweet victory is mine!

Strategize what you will need to get what you want. Be committed and productive, so you can see results.

3. PLANT: Plant a seed of change. You have the power to make change happen. When you fail to change, you repeat the same habits and end up with the same results. Sow good seeds into your health so that you can reap a strong harvest.

4. HAVE FAITH: Use your faith to serve as your foundation, your rock. Take dominion over your mental, spiritual, and physical being. You can't compromise, negotiate, or waiver in your faith when it comes to your health. Gospel singer Mahalia Jackson once said, "Faith and prayer are the vitamins of the soul. Man cannot live in health without them."

Now, you may have to run through these breaking-free strategies every day until you are truly walking in total freedom. Just know that with each step you take down that path of promise, it's worth it! You're worth it! Remember, you are stronger than any stronghold!

3

Putting the Power in Willpower

'm starting with the man in the mirror. I'm asking him to change his ways." Michael Jackson sang those powerful words. If you're going to have success in your life, you have to live those words. In order to increase your willpower, create new habits, envision a new you, and actually become the person you were created to be, you must commit to changing your ways. You have to look at your reflection in the mirror and say, "It's time to make a change."

Change starts internally, not externally. If you want something different, you have to do something different. Change is necessary in moving forward, but you have to want to change more than you want to stay the same. Remember, your mindset and your faith have to be of one accord so that you can have the power to make change happen.

That's what Brenda Anderson had to do, but once she decided to make the necessary changes to achieve a strong, healthy body, the weight came off. When Brenda held up the jeans that had fit her snugly just nine months before, tears welled up in her eyes. She could almost fit into one leg of those old jeans. After taking a step of faith and joining a club for fitness at her church, Brenda continued to

steadily lose pounds and inches. Her goal: to lose a total of 125 pounds in one calendar year. Not only did Brenda successfully lose all that weight, but she also gained the self-confidence and self-esteem she never dreamed were possible. She feels empowered and excited about her future. "I am a new person on the inside and the outside," she says. "Before I lost the weight, I would just try to blend into the background of life. I didn't want anyone to notice me. But not now."

Today, she is a fitness coach at her Chicago-area church, helping others accomplish their dreams. In fact, she has so much self-confidence that she just filmed a video testimonial, sharing her fitness transformation. "I love talking to people now," she says. "I love being an example and sharing my

SWEET TWEET

Praise is my weapon, for the only begotten Risen Son!

God created us all 2 a specific call; the one who is against U & me will surely fall.

story, and I fully expect that my testimony will impact other people's lives."

From wallflower to wildfire, from feeling pitiful to being powerful—that's our Miss Brenda. Romans 2:11 tells us that God is no respecter of persons, but what he did for Brenda, he will do for you, if you will only decide to make those necessary changes and find that power within to conquer each goal. You have the power within yourself to move forward. Change happens on the inside before it manifests itself on the outside. Although Brenda was more than 125 pounds from her goal weight when she started, she trusted in her faith and had the courage, confidence, and commitment to make it happen. So say out loud, "I'm full of power, and this is my hour!"

Set Goals! W2Fit Cards!

Now that you're fired up to go for your dreams, here are some practical tips that will empower you. How do you achieve your goals? It's about setting goals that are definite, achievable, measurable, and significant:

DEFINITE: specific and precise

ACHIEVABLE: attainable

MEASURABLE: accountable and timely

SIGNIFICANT: meaningful

A goal that has the above characteristics will help you break old habits and obtain new habits so you can be successful. For example, one of my goals is to have daily devotion for thirty to sixty minutes, which includes meditation and prayer, so I can nourish and strengthen my spiritual being. To help me stay focused and reach my goals, I use Witness to Fitness goal cards, better known as W2Fit cards. I list my goals on the cards, decorate them, and at the bottom of each I write, "It's Possible." I post my W2Fit cards on my mirror in my bathroom, carry them in my purse or briefcase, and keep them on my desk, so I can always have with me my vision of what I will accomplish. W2Fit cards are daily reminders of me being a witness to my faith, family, purpose, and passion.

To help you accomplish your ideal weight, write down a goal on a W2Fit card. Then go to www.health status.com/calculate/ideal-healthy-weight online and plug in your height and sex. It will give you a healthy weight range and an ideal target weight. Instead of just saying, "I need to lose some weight," you now have a specific goal weight in mind. Brenda Anderson found out her goal weight and worked toward achieving it.

As a general rule, I advocate gradual weight loss over anything too drastic. Sure, you may lose weight quickly with a liquid or an extreme diet, but these programs slow down your metabolism and leave you with only temporary weight loss. Once you start eating regular food again, you'll likely put the weight right back on and become discouraged. The idea here is to develop new habits so you can maintain your new weight.

It also helps to set short-term goals, then reward yourself each time you achieve one. That's what Brenda did. When she joined the fitness club at her church, she wanted to drop a specific amount of weight by her thirty-year high school reunion six months later, and she did! With every milestone she hit, Brenda bought herself a new outfit, which served two purposes: it was a reward for her hard work and it gave her new clothes to show off her beautiful body. Celebrate the little victories along the way. Those mini celebrations will motivate you to stay on track until you reach your ultimate goal.

Telling Your Story / Journaling

Journaling is not just a good idea; it's a God idea. Habakkuk 2:2 says to write the vision and make it plain so you can run with it. Even if you've never liked the idea of journaling, think of it as just telling your story. Write down your goals, visions, accomplishments, thoughts, and so on, and be honest and real.

Why is this important to do? Journaling, or telling your story, empowers you, provides focus and clarity, and improves your psychological well-being. It's also a perfect way to enhance your spiritual health by writing about your connection to God. There are no rules for what you write or how you record your thoughts. You could create a personal blog, record your voice, record a video, or simply write in a notebook. I record my experiences more now than ever before, because as I mature, my memory isn't as sharp as it used to be. I tell my story in my journal and I get energized, because it's a reminder of how much closer I am to realizing my dreams. I tell my story by sharing my thoughts, goals, progress, accomplishments, and even prayers.

Telling your story also provides you with an outlet to remind yourself of God's grace and goodness. Often I will thank him for accompanying me on my path and giving me the vision to see what he has called me to do. So write the vision, tell your story, and be a witness!

Looking Forward

This chapter is about power, and let me be real—there is no power if all your energy is focused on your past. Trying to live in the past, or continuing to dwell in past thoughts, will keep you from the future. It's time to look forward, not backward. Why do you think the front windshield of your car is so much larger than the rearview mirror? Because you're supposed to be spending most of your time looking forward, not backward.

At some point in the process, you have to make a decision that you're not turning back. I had to make that decision when I hiked up Mount Kilimanjaro. We were almost to the midway point of the trek when we came to a steep wall. I studied it, and then asked our guide, "Is there a way around this wall?" He smiled and said, "No, we're going to scale it." I started surveying the situation and then noticed that nowhere in our stash of goodies was a harness belt or any kind of scaling equipment. It was do or die, literally! Since this was such a monumental decision, I knew that all of us had to be in agreement concerning our next move, so we prayed. At the end of that prayer session, we unanimously decided to go for it. That was a defining moment. We were each declaring, "I am doing this, and there is no turning back!" As I scaled that steep wall, I didn't look down. I didn't look back. I just kept pressing onward and upward. And that's

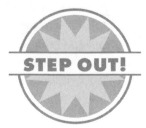

Remember to create your W2Fit cards so you can always see that your goals are within reach. Along the way, tell your story by journaling your experience of transforming your health and your life. "For nothing is impossible with God" (Luke 1:37).

exactly what you have to do when you face any mountain in your life: you have to charge forward, reminding yourself that where there is a will, you make a way.

Steven Curtis Chapman's song "Burn the Ships" really captures this truth. The song tells the story of Cortés and his Spanish fleet and the mission they embarked on in 1519. Of course, as you probably remember from eighth-grade history, they landed on the eastern shore of Mexico with big plans, but the New World was very hard and they became discouraged. They wanted to go back home to the comfortable life they knew. But as Cortés tells them, "Burn the ships. We're here to stay."

I'm telling you today: let the ships burn. You've passed the point of no return! You've come too far on this journey to turn back now. Instead, focus on what the new you will look like and how the new you will feel. Look to the future! Think about how much you've accomplished so far. Even if you haven't lost a pound, the fact that you picked up this book and have read this far proves that you're serious about making a change and moving ahead.

Looking back can be so dangerous. You look back with longing, wishing you could return to

that place, to that time, in that body. When I ask people about their health goals, they often pull out a picture of themselves from twenty years ago. If it's been twenty years since that picture was snapped, your body has changed and your metabolism has slowed down. You can't be who you were and who you are at the same time. Work with what you have, to be the best you can be.

I have a colleague who is very fit and has maintained a high level of fitness for many years, so I was surprised when she expressed to me her frustration with her body. She said she had set a goal to achieve the weight she was in college, which was about thirty years ago. I asked, "Did you do it?" She replied, "Yeah, I was down to that weight after much work . . . but I couldn't stay there." I smiled at her and said, "Hey, it's admirable that you set that goal and met it, but it might be impossible to maintain an unrealistic goal. Give yourself a break! How far are you over that college weight today?" She answered, "Only 5 pounds. I've been able to maintain that weight." I congratulated her on that success and told her to celebrate instead of being so hard on herself. At that moment it was as if a huge burden had been lifted off of her. She smiled and said, "I have been trying to be who I was and not who I am today. I can't be both."

My colleague is not unlike most of us. We all have that dream weight that we wish we still were, or a pair of jeans we wore in college that we hope to fit into again someday, but those are not realistic goals. The truth is, things in your life have changed, and your body definitely has changed. Your look may be different because your body may have spread, increased, drooped, or puckered. Think of yourself as a car. When you drove that car off the lot new, it didn't have a scratch on it. It was a fine machine. But over the years you've probably had to do some repairs and upkeep on that vehicle, right? Well, your body is the same way. You've got more miles on you now, and even with the proper upkeep and bodywork, you'll never look quite the same way as you did when you were younger, and that's okay. By desiring to look like that picture again, you're setting yourself up for failure. You're actually trying to fit into the old you. Look forward to the new you. Get a new vision and stop looking behind. Nothing good ever comes from dwelling in the past. Remember, your power isn't in the past; it's in your present and your future.

From Setback to Setup

To step into this new life, you can't keep doing the same old same old. That keeps you at the status quo, and that's not the goal, right? But incorporating new habits isn't always easy. You will probably encounter setbacks along the path to better health; just don't let your circumstances discourage you from moving forward.

Think of it like this: a setback is a setup for a comeback. When a setback happens, there's a tendency to say, "I've tried working out and eating better, but I just can't stick to it." Once you skip a week of working out or give in to eating a pint of ice cream, it's easy to let those miscues define you or discourage you from getting back on the wagon and finishing your course. But you can't allow temporary circumstances to hinder your progress. See them as that—an interruption. So what? You had a lapse in your program. Forgive yourself and move ahead. Yesterday is gone forever; today is a new day with a fresh start. Lamentations 3:23 says that God's mercies are new every morning, so embrace those new mercies and move on!

I know this isn't going to be easy. But there is no success without struggle. There is no testimony

without a test. There is no victory without a fight. Biblically speaking, you can't get to the Promised Land before you've gone through the wilderness. But your wilderness time is over! You have the power within you to succeed.

As you progress toward good health, people will start noticing changes in you. Maybe you have more energy than before. Maybe you're not eating as much fried food as you used to, or you're walking during your lunch hour instead of going out to eat with coworkers. Perhaps you're even buying new clothes in smaller sizes and exuding a new confidence. You're in the midst of transformation from the old you to the new you. You feel different and you act differently. These changes aren't surprising. After all, you're facing challenges and conquering them one by one. Of course you feel empowered. Think of your journey as climbing a mountain. As you progress up that mountain, you feel energized, strong, and proud. You're keeping

TRANSFORMATION *Tidbits*

- It's time to set goals that are definite, achievable, measurable, and significant.

- A setback is a setup for a comeback.

- "You must eat from the garden of your own thoughts, so don't grow anything you don't want to eat." —Bishop T. D. Jakes

- You're in the midst of transforming from the old you to the new you.

- Remember, what's in front of you is much more powerful than what's behind you.

- Find the rhythm of your well-being and begin moving to the groove of your new life.

the ultimate goal in mind with every step you take. No matter how difficult the journey, you keep that goal before you.

That's what I had to do. As I climbed Mount Kilimanjaro, I envisioned myself at the top of it, giving thanks and doing a front flip. Any negative thoughts that entered my mind during my climb were immediately discarded. I had planted the seeds of positive thoughts during my weeks of preparation, and those seeds grew into a full-blown garden of positivity. I didn't have room for any stinkin' thinkin' weeds in my garden. My pastor, Bishop T. D. Jakes, once said, "You must eat from the garden of your own thoughts, so don't grow anything you don't want to eat." Chew on that for a moment. While climbing up the steep terrain, I thought only about conquering that mountain. It was a constant battle—nine days of working the plan to get to the top—but I stayed focused on the ultimate goal. With each small step, my belief in myself and in my Creator grew stronger. Quitting simply wasn't an option. At one point we met up with some other hikers, and one of them took a look at me and my team, gave me a little smirk, and said, "Good luck." Without missing a beat, I answered, "What does luck have to do with it? You better know Jesus!"

No matter what challenge you're facing today—a 100-pound weight-loss goal, an illness, or an emotional wound—you'd better have a higher source to pull from. I always joke with my friends, "You better put on your big girl panties." But I am telling you, when I conquered Mount Kilimanjaro, I had to put on my Jesus drawers. And you'll have to do the same if you're going to make the changes to the person in the mirror that are necessary to move toward good health, healing, and happiness. You have to have strength, tenacity, and guts to conquer your mountain, but you can do it!

The New You

Some people will abandon you on your mission. Others will speak negatively about you. And after you've accomplished your goal, not everyone will be ready to celebrate with you. When I returned from my climb up Kilimanjaro, some folks didn't act the same toward me. Looking back, I'm not surprised, because *I* was different. Climbing that mountain changed me forever. I climbed up and down steep slopes carrying a forty-pound backpack. I encountered eighty-nine-degree temperatures at the bottom of the mountain and below-zero temperatures at the summit. At times, I was gasping for every breath, because the air was thin and my body had to work harder. I slept in a sleeping bag on the ground, and I wasn't able to shower for nine straight days. (Thank God for wet wipes.) I had to use the great outdoors as my toilet, and when I ran out of toilet paper, I made do with leaves. And when "Aunt Flo" came to visit unexpectedly, I had to use T-shirts, toilet paper, and duct tape to get me through. It was rough. That mountain, the terrain, the climate, and the wilderness itself presented constant challenges. But then there were the moments like when I was trekking at 17,000 feet with the clouds below me. It was simply beautiful and surreal.

After struggling through those experiences and ultimately accomplishing my goal, I came home with more courage, strength, and wisdom. I felt transformed and people noticed. Some people embraced the new me, but others kept looking for the old Donna. The problem was, the old Donna was still on that mountain. I had left her there and returned with a new-and-improved version of myself. I couldn't help it if some of my friends weren't ready for her. Your friends and family may have a hard time letting go of the old you, but resist the pressure to return to that old self.

It may feel good to eat the same fattening foods the old you once consumed. It may feel comfortable to skip your workout and hang out with friends and family. You may have temptations, but put the *power* in willpower and stay true to who you are now. Invite your friends and family to join you. Challenge them to move their bodies more, eat healthy foods, and embrace this new way of living too. If they won't accompany you, do it anyway—even if it means making the trek alone.

Stay on track and don't look back! Stop trying to please the people in your life. Focus on what's best for you. In the end, many people will respect you, and you might even inspire them to reach for a higher level of newness in their own health.

Remember, what's in front of you is much more powerful than what's behind you. Let yourself evolve instead of staying the same, so you can be better than ever before. As you look into the future, create new habits and envision the new you. Find the rhythm of your well-being and begin moving to the groove of your new life.

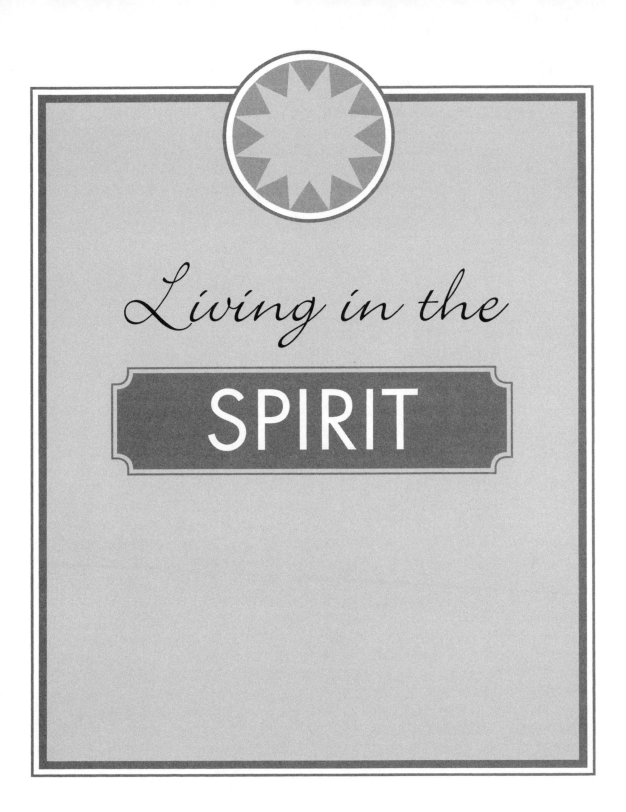

Living in the

SPIRIT

The Fab Four Formula

The world's view of health focuses more on the external instead of the internal components. I see it differently. When teaching about total health, you have to think it, believe it, and act on it. That's why we're approaching your total health from a mind, spirit, and body perspective. You should have a new mind-set, after reading the past three chapters. Now we're ready to align your thought processes and find that inner strength, so that you can act on your new mind-set—the spirit aspect. We'll cover fitness and nutrition in chapters 7 and 8—the body aspect. By the time you've read the last word of this book, you'll be ready to walk in total health and wholeness, and be a witness to fitness.

The Fab Four

Whenever I coach people concerning their spiritual health, I share four crucial aspects I call the Fab Four: vision, faith, passion, and purpose. When you have all four working for you, success is inevitable.

VISION

Helen Keller once said, "The only thing worse than being blind is having sight but no vision." Proverbs 29:18 says, "Where there is no vision, the people perish." And I say, "Your vision is the imagination and inspiration for where you want to go." Where do you want to go?

The first step is to write down your vision. Figure out what you want out of life, and make sure it is your Creator's plan. Once you have a sense of your purpose, your vision statement should be easy to write. A vision statement is simply an idealized, detailed description of a desired outcome, which inspires and invigorates you to press toward your

---

SWEET TWEET

Don't sit around & be down.
Pick up! Get up! Clean up!

U have a race 2 finish. Evacuate anything
that will hinder your growth or diminish.

goal. Your vision statement should be so specific and emotionally charged that it creates a mental picture of that desired outcome. For example, I once read that Microsoft's vision statement in the 1980s was simply, "A personal computer in every home running Microsoft software." It's very short, to the point, and clear. And it focuses everyone on the big picture.

Don't stop at a vision statement. Take the next step and create your own vision tree.

Vision Tree

To help you stay focused on your greater assignments, I created a vision tree, which is similar to a vision board. A vision board helps you focus with clarity and gives you a picture of your goals. Images and words on the board represent the goals you strive for. A vision tree does the same thing, except it digs a little deeper.

Every tree has a root system. "We should be rooted in God, who is the ground of our being," says Marcia Hollis. The parts of a tree you see are the trunk, branches, and leaves; the part you don't see is the root system. With us, there is our physical being—our bodies, our words, and our actions, which are seen and heard, and our minds and spirits, which are not seen. Like a tree, if we have strong roots, we can weather a storm, because our roots are deep enough to keep us steadfast in our faith. The roots of a tree have to grow deep to provide nourishment and strength so the tree can survive bad conditions; otherwise, it will be destroyed. Be rooted, like a strong fruit tree. Its branches bear the weight of the fruit, its leaves gather nourishment and stimulate new growth, its fruit is the evidence of productivity, and the seeds from the fruit give birth to reproduction. Imagine your vision tree representing your life and the fruits of your labor. Your foundation in God feeds and nourishes your total well-being

and helps you to continue to grow. Trees need sunshine and rain. We need God's love and mercy. "Christ may dwell in your hearts through faith, as you are being rooted and grounded in love" (Eph. 3:17). The benefit of having and evolving your vision tree is similar to a family tree or a tree of life; you are nurturing your vision of building a tree for generations to come.

What are your roots grounded in? What gives you strength in life? How do you plan to be more fruitful in your life? Every day you are sowing your vision. You're either sowing good seeds or bad seeds, but you're always planting something. If you're sowing seeds of hope, determination, and perseverance, your harvest will be a good one. But if you're sowing seeds of doubt, negativity, and fear, your crops won't be worth harvesting. You need to water the seeds of hope in your vision tree. Don't allow those weeds of negativity to creep into your vision tree and choke your dreams. Refuse to let negative thoughts overtake your blessings. Tell yourself, "I will do whatever it takes to accomplish my vision." Having the courage and faith in your spirit will turn a negative into a positive, a wrong into a right, an "I can't" into an "I can." Your purpose in life will become all too clear—just like it did for Bethany Hamilton.

A few years ago only those in the surfing world knew the name Bethany Hamilton. She had been surfing since she was eleven years old and was considered a rising star in her sport. At thirteen, she was already competing against older girls and women in amateur events, and beating many of them. She was definitely on her way to turning professional—but the unthinkable happened. On an October morning in 2003, thirteen-year-old Bethany Hamilton hit the waves at Tunnels Beach in Kauai, Hawaii, with several of her friends and two strong arms. A few hours later, a 14-foot tiger shark tore Bethany's left arm from her body.

Somehow, Bethany managed to paddle her way to shore, and even though she had lost a lot of blood, she miraculously survived.

In the weeks and months that followed, she had to learn how to live with only one arm. She had to get a new vision statement and push toward a new dream. Sure, she could've given up or been angry at her Creator, but Bethany did just the opposite. She turned her tragedy into a triumph and started surfing again. In fact, she was named ESPY's Best Comeback Athlete in 2004. Plus, Bethany found that her story gave her a platform to share her testimony of faith. She wrote a book called *Soul Surfer: A True Story of Faith, Family, and Fighting to Get Back on the Board,* and in 2011 her story was made into a major motion picture, which is inspiring people all over the world to fight back and chase after their dreams, no matter what.

So are you letting your tests become testimonies? Don't let obstacles—no matter how big they may seem—block your vision. If you encounter the unexpected, keep pressing through to glory. Remember, "Success is intentional; failure is not an option!"

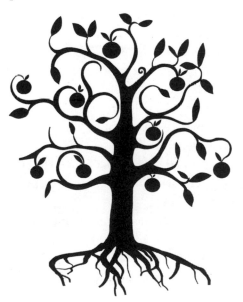

FAITH

If you desire to improve your well-being and live life to the fullest, start by increasing your faith. Faith is defined in the dictionary as a belief in God or in the doctrines and teachings of a religion. Your belief system holds you accountable to the morals and values in your life. God wants us not to just study the word but to apply it to our lives. Faith is about having a relationship with God, or a greater source, and knowing he is the ultimate source. The Creator expects us to have discipline in our thoughts and actions, because he is the foundation of our beings.

As you grow spiritually, your faith is woven into the fabric of your being and prayer becomes an integral part of your daily life. I start my day with meditation, which is focused on calming my mind and listening to God. Prayer is my talk, my praise, and my worship with him. This book is about faith and fitness, and you're the caretaker of your body, which is the temple of the Holy Spirit. Do you treasure or trash your temple? Do you treat it with reverence and respect?

Your journey is not just physical but spiritual, mental, and emotional. Every facet of your life should be centered around your faith. "Faith is the substance of things hoped for, the evidence of things not seen" (Heb. 11:1). We must be rooted in our faith, so the breath of God gives us energy to grow and evolve. Because your mind, spirit, and body are interconnected, the health of one affects the health of the others. Some people focus on one and not the others, but you must trust in your greater source for all, so that you can have a better sense of self and purpose.

I remember a time when I didn't have a strong relationship with God, and my life was out of control. During that time I didn't have strong principles to follow and I didn't have self-love and inner peace. I believed it but I didn't live it. In retrospect, it's only because of his goodness and grace that I made it through. When I put him first, all aspects of my life changed, and I learned to decrease self and increase him.

Whether you are Jewish, Christian, or Muslim, your faith is tied to something greater than you, and that union will carry you through life's sweet and sour times. Oscar Wilde once said, "To live is the rarest thing in the world. Most people exist, that is all." I believe we were put on this earth to grow into the persons we were created to be.

With a deeply rooted faith, you can accomplish anything. That's what Stephanie discovered when she began my fitness program. She knew that God had called her to mentor the young women in her local church, but she didn't feel like she was setting a good example for them in the physical realm. So she set out to lose weight, get fit, and become a witness for fitness. She realized that her calling, her destiny, and her ultimate purpose in life could not be fulfilled to the best of her ability without making some changes in her lifestyle. Once she let her faith motivate her, Stephanie became the role model she always wanted to be.

When Dawn, who lost more than 240 pounds following my program, started the program to improve herself, she soon discovered that her journey was twofold. It wasn't just about getting fit for herself personally but being a living example for her child too. Her son, who had been diagnosed as borderline obese, has since gone from couch potato to athlete. In fact, he is excelling in both academics and athletics. Dawn says her faith has everything to do with her own success as well as her son's. Although she is excited about her weight loss, it does not compare to how she has grown spiritually. I feel blessed to have had the opportunity to help Dawn. What makes me even more proud of her is how she is helping others.

PASSION

Passion is the third aspect of my Fab Four formula for success. If there's one thing I know about passion, it's that it requires participation. In other words, you have to think it, believe it, and act on it. You have to believe your goals are possible and use your passion to fuel your pursuit of them. Your attitude has to be "yes, I can" followed by "yes, I did." Your passion is the connector between those two states of being.

You may be at a point in your life when you are ready to embrace change, or you may not be there yet. When you finally feel enough is enough, you'll get serious about reaching your goal. The power to change is within you, but you have to activate that power with passion.

Passion is defined as a strong liking or desire for or devotion to some activity, object, or concept. It's the driving life force that keeps you in the game when you would rather quit and sit on the side-

BONNAMITE SOUND BITE

You need faith for this journey because life can be tough. But, honey, you've got God, who is more than enough!

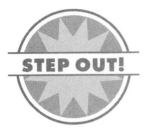

lines. You will need that kind of passion to achieve your purpose and destiny.

Passion helps us do what seems impossible. Just ask J. R. Martinez, who won the thirteenth season title on *Dancing with the Stars* alongside pro partner Karina Smirnoff. Martinez, an Iraq veteran, suffered severe burns over 40 percent of his body when the Humvee he was driving hit a land mine in April 2003, but he proved that nothing is impossible if you have the passion to pursue your dreams. According to *USA Today*, after winning the much-celebrated dancing competition, Martinez kissed his mother and said, "Can you believe that eight and a half years ago you were teaching me how to walk?"

It was a long journey from Martinez's injury to his win on *Dancing with the Stars*. He spent thirty-four months in recovery at Brooke Army Medical Center in San Antonio, Texas, where he endured thirty-three different surgeries. He didn't spend his days in recovery feeling sorry for himself, though; instead, he shared his story with other patients at the hospital and encouraged them. His passion to serve hadn't ended in that Humvee in Iraq. It carried over into his new life, and he was serving others any way that he could. His remarkable spirit gained the attention of others, and soon he was making appearances on *Oprah, 60 Minutes,* CNN, and more. Since 2004, Martinez has been touring the nation with his message of hope. In 2008 Martinez even joined the cast of ABC's day-time drama *All My Children* as combat veteran character Brot Monroe. After the *Dancing with the Stars* finale, a grateful and fulfilled Martinez said, "I just want to breathe and take it all in. It's been such an amazing journey."

But that experience never would have begun if Martinez hadn't possessed the passion to take that first step. Let your passion be your driving force. Start the ignition and take off.

PURPOSE

The fourth component of my Fab Four formula is purpose. Purpose is defined as something set up as an object or an end to be attained. Think about what your purpose is in your health and your life. We just discussed passion, which leads you to your purpose. You have to think, believe, and act on purpose. You can't stay in your comfort zone, if you're living on purpose.

Once I faced one of the greatest challenges in my life and it broke me down, and I mean all the way down. Yet I didn't allow my pain to stop my passion. My pain fueled my passion, which in turn ignited my purpose. At times I felt my burning desire was being smothered, and I felt despair, but something in my soul continued to push me to realize my dreams, despite adversity. I was knocked down, but I was not out. I had to look up, not down.

I had to be steadfast in my purpose, just like fitness pioneer Jack LaLanne. In 1951, decades

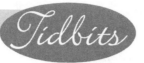
TRANSFORMATION *Tidbits*

- You have to think it, believe it, and act on it.

- When you have vision, faith, passion, and purpose working for you, success is inevitable.

- When your faith is rooted in a higher source, you have strength beyond yourself.

- A vision tree inspires and invigorates you to press toward your goals.

- You have to believe your goals are possible and use your passion to fuel your pursuit.

---

before Richard Simmons and Jane Fonda popularized the concept, Jack LaLanne's TV show introduced physical fitness to millions of Americans. He's now referred to as the "godfather of fitness" because he essentially started the fitness and health industry.

Jack described himself in his teens as a sugarholic junk-food junkie, and he openly admitted he'd had behavioral problems, but at age fifteen his life took a different turn. After he listened to a lecture by Paul Bragg, a well-known nutritionist, he became a fitness and health advocate and began a movement. He believed that the overall health of our country's population needed improvement.

Jack spread the gospel of good health by promoting daily physical activity and good nutrition. His TV show, which I watched along with those millions of others, was a big hit up until the time it was taken off the air. (It was replaced with *The Today Show,* which I was blessed to work on for several years as a fitness expert.) Jack opened one of the first gyms in America, in Oakland, California, and it became a model for other gyms. His heart was bigger than life. He wanted to help all people, so he started coaching the elderly and physically challenged too. At the age of fifty-four he was still going strong and beat Arnold Schwarzenegger, then twenty-one, in an unofficial bodybuilding contest. Beat the Speedos off him.

Although Jack LaLanne is no longer with us, I did have the opportunity to thank him for pioneering the fitness and health industry I now proudly serve. Jack lived and served with purpose! When you use the Fab Four: vision, faith, passion, and purpose you can live exceedingly and abundantly, beyond all you could ever imagine.

5

You're Closer Than You Think

When Hee Kyung Seo, the 2011 Louise Suggs Rolex Rookie of the Year winner, gave her speech at the LPGA event, she wowed the whole room with her words of wisdom and encouragement. She expressed the importance of praising the higher source in our lives. She urged everyone to keep a grateful heart, even when things don't go as planned. And she shared how she always tries to be thankful for the small victories on the way to a major goal. Then she said something I'll never forget. I wanted to run up on stage and high-five her. She spoke about Yani Tseng as someone she looks up to in the golf world, because Yani has accomplished so much in her twenty-two years of life. In fact, when Yani won the Ricoh Women's British Open, she became the youngest golfer ever to claim five major championships. After listing all of Yani's many feats, Hee added, "And Yani, I'm coming for you. You know when you're driving your car and your mirror says OBJECTS MAY BE CLOSER THAN YOU THINK? Well, that will be me."

I love that! You see, every step we take is one step closer to victory. Sure, there will be times when your goals seem too difficult to achieve or too far off, but you just might be closer than you think. Hebrews 10:35 says, "Don't get discouraged; payday is coming." My mother always said, "It's darkest before the dawn." I've found that to be true in life. Sometimes life seems the hardest when that breakthrough is right around the corner. At that point, the naysayers in your life will try to get you to quit. Self-doubt and discouragement will arise, but don't allow these to take over. Say, "I've come too far to stop now." Tell your naysayers, "Do what you may, I choose to pray!"

I once heard Joel Osteen, pastor of Lakewood Church, share a story about hiking up a mountain

SWEET TWEET

We live in a world that spins around & around. U are sharp, smart, & resilient, so don't wear a frown.

Naysayers do what U may.
I choose 2 pray.

in Colorado, which speaks to this truth of being closer than you think. I could relate to every word he spoke. Pastor Joel recounted that a sign at the bottom of the mountain indicated that the hike to the top would take about three hours and the elevation was about 11,000 feet above sea level. Now, Joel is a runner, so he was in shape for this hike, yet he found himself feeling winded after only forty-five minutes. His legs were burning. He was sweating. When he rested for a moment, thinking about turning back, he encountered an older gentleman coming down the mountain. That older man looked at Joel, smiled, and said, "You are closer than you think." That one phrase gave Joel the second wind he needed to push forward, and sure enough, just ten minutes later, he reached the top of that mountain. The hike had only taken him one hour—not three, like the sign at the base of the mountain had said. Without that older man's words of encouragement, he might have given up. Joel had thought he had two more hours of difficult hiking at that point but, in actuality, he'd had only ten more minutes to endure before reaching his goal.

I wonder how many times in life we're closer to achieving our goals than we think, and yet we give up because we can't see the finish line? How many times do we throw in the towel and settle right where we are because we're afraid we won't be able to finish strong? Too many people get weary on their paths and, instead of pushing through their pain, they quit before they cross the finish line.

That makes me think of a story shared by Chip Brim, author of *Are You a Champion 4 Christ?* He had a dream one night, and what he saw made him very sad. Chip described a football field with many people running toward the end zone. Chip was like the ultimate fan, cheering them on to victory, but when they arrived at the one-yard line, they all stopped. Not a single one of them made it into the end zone. He said it was such a troubling image that he sought God about it, and God gave him insight into the dream. God showed him that those people running for the end zone are like many of us. We start off strong, running with heart and passion, but when we get close enough to taste victory, we quit. We run out of gas. We give up. The Creator was sharing with Chip that it was time to finish what we start. It's time to go after those dreams with everything in us and refuse to quit—no matter what.

I've found that there comes a point when that supernatural force wells up inside you and causes you to face your Goliath once and for all. That's when you look your Goliath right in the eye and declare, "You're not taking me down. I'm taking you down! I'll be the last one standing."

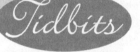

TRANSFORMATION *Tidbits*

- Every step you take is one step closer to victory.
- Sometimes life seems the hardest when a breakthrough is right around the corner, but stay the course.
- Tell your naysayers, "Do what you may, I choose to pray!"
- Use your tough times to catapult you from a state of comfort to your ultimate victory.
- "Thoughts form attitudes and attitudes determine destiny."—Bishop Dennis Leonard
- It's time to trust God in every area of your life, including your mental, spiritual, and physical health.

Never Would Have Made It

That's what pastor and songwriter Marvin Sapp had to do when he was going through one of the darkest times in his life—the death of his father. He had buried his dad a few days before and was in the pulpit, ready to deliver a message to his congregation when he heard the spirit of God tell him, "Marvin, there's something you need to understand. Although your father isn't with you physically, I will never leave you. Nor will I forsake you. I will be with you always, even until the end of the earth." At that moment, Marvin gave birth to the award-winning song "Never Would Have Made It." He grabbed the microphone and started singing, "Never would have made it, never could have made it, without you." When you face challenging times, this song will help comfort and heal you.

Don't give up during the tough times. Use those experiences to press forward in your future. Your pain has purpose, so let it be the fuel to move you ahead. Your tough times can catapult you from a state of comfort to your ultimate victory. Your job

is this: don't sink into despair! Work that thing out, and work that thing through. Be thankful, even in the most difficult times, because this too shall pass.

Focus on Your Future

Romans 8:28 says, "And we know that all things work together for the good of them that love God, to them who are called according to his purpose." "All things" means all things, right? That means even when your get-up-and-go has got up and gone. When you feel like you're down for the count, don't count yourself out! You can rest in the fact that your faith will carry you through. Think about how far you've come, not how much farther you have to go. The way you think determines the way you feel, and the way you feel determines the way you act. So put your thoughts in check.

I like that Kodak slogan, "Celebrate the moments of your life." We need to take time to celebrate the little things in life. When we do this, we leave no time for dwelling on the bad memories or

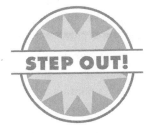

"A smile costs nothing but gives much. It enriches those who receive without making poorer those who give. It takes but a moment, but the memory of it sometimes lasts forever. None is so rich or mighty that he cannot get along without it, and none is so poor that he cannot be made rich by it. Yet a smile cannot be bought, begged, borrowed, or stolen, for it is something that is of no value to anyone until it is given away. Some people are too tired to give you a smile. Give them one of yours, as none needs a smile as much as he who has no more to give."

—Anonymous

I challenge you to share a smile everywhere you go today. Just putting a smile on your face will improve your attitude and the attitudes of those around you.

difficult times that once plagued us. No, all our energies are tied up in celebrating the day-to-day victories and meditating on the magical moments. That's a much happier place to live.

Think about looking through your family photo albums. Every picture captures a moment with relatives smiling at one another, friends embracing, children laughing and playing, etc. We don't include pictures of siblings fighting or photos of us lying in bed with our heads buried beneath the covers. Why? Because we don't want to remember those times. We want to recall happy, wonderful memories. Treat your mind like a photo album and choose not to store unhappy pictures; only allow happy images of joyful times to remain in your mind and spirit. Dwelling in the past—good or bad—is not productive. Stay focused on what's ahead of you, not what's behind you.

Take it from Lot's wife: looking back is not beneficial to your future. You probably remember that Bible story. God sent his angels to Sodom and Gomorrah to observe the cities' wickedness firsthand. After they had seen enough, the angels took Lot, his wife, and their daughters away from the cities to save them, because God had decided to destroy Sodom and Gomorrah. But as they left the

evil cities, Lot's wife looked behind her with longing. Sure, the cities were evil, but they had been her home and she wanted to dwell there in her mind one last time. When she disobediently looked behind her, God immediately turned her into a pillar of salt. So what's the lesson here? When God is trying to do a new thing in your life and propel you forward, don't look back and long for your past. It is not about your plan but about God's plans for your life. Focus on your future!

Make the Right Choice

In his book *Happiness Matters: 21 Thoughts That Could Change Your Life,* Bishop Dennis Leonard writes, "If you get your thinking right and keep a good attitude, happiness will come into your life and stay in your life. When you think positively, you have a positive attitude, and as a result your whole life will have a positive charge. . . . Thoughts form attitudes and attitudes determine destiny."

Guinness world record holder Ernestine Shepherd can say amen to that statement. At age fifty-six she changed her attitude about healthy living and went from hardly moving to becoming a mover and a shaker in the health and fitness world. From fitness training to competitive bodybuilding, Ernestine has accomplished much in the past twenty years—including gaining the Guinness world title as the oldest competitive female bodybuilder—and she's inspired many along the way.

"I am a seventy-five-year-old woman," she told *Hope for Women* magazine in December 2011. "I don't want to be defined by my shape or size or by my personal strength. What matters to me is living a healthy, happy, positive, confident lifestyle, and to pass this on to others."

It all began with a change in attitude. After trying on bathing suits, she and her sister decided

BONNAMITE SOUND BITE

Show the world your big, cheesy grin because you know you shine from within!

they needed to improve their bodies, and the two middle-aged women committed themselves to improving their health. Almost immediately, the dynamic duo began doing aerobics. Their instructor suggested the siblings also incorporate weightlifting into their weekly workouts. Ernestine fought it at first, but after seeing results, she embraced strength training. However, that wasn't enough. The sisters knew that if they wanted to see dramatic results, they would need to start eating healthy too, so they did.

Unfortunately, Ernestine's sister died unexpectedly of a brain aneurysm, leaving Ernestine to chase after the dream of a strong, fit body all by herself. At first, she didn't want to pursue it alone. She stopped exercising and eating right and ended up with high blood pressure, panic attacks, acid reflux, and depression. But this setback was really a setup for success. Eventually, she got up out of her depressed state and started again. "I decided I was going to follow the dream my sister and I had," she said.

Her new mantra became: Determined, Dedicated, and Disciplined to be fit. She lives those three Ds every day, and she tells the people she trains that they have to do the same. Ernestine is a living example that it's never too late to change your attitude and your destiny. When asked what she hopes for most in life, she responded, "I hope that within my lifetime it will go down that I have helped people to know that you only have one life, and to live it as healthy as you possibly can. Don't let anyone ever tell you that you cannot."

The Ds Equal Victories

That's good advice for all of us. Don't let the haters keep you from achieving your dreams. Don't let setbacks stop your progress. Keep your eye on your goals and remember that you just might be closer than you think! Sure, you're going to come up against some challenges, but your foundation of faith makes you unshakable. When you build your entire life on faith, you won't waver, compromise, or be moved! I meet people all the time who have faith in God, but when it comes to their health they leave faith out of the equation. This thought process leaves me baffled. If you trust in a higher source for everything else in your life, then why don't you trust him with your health and well-being? It's time to put your faith into action. That includes your mental, spiritual, and physical health. Start right where you are and take Ernestine's advice: be determined, dedicated, and disciplined. And let me add a few more Ds—be deliberate and be a dreamer. These Ds will result in big victories in your life if you'll live them every day. Celebrate today, realizing that you're closer than you think.

6

Move to Give

When people first meet my family, they are usually surprised. It seems perfectly normal for us to share a yummy meal, push the tables and chairs out of the way, turn on the music, and start dancing. Apparently this is not the norm, but you know what? It should be! We should not be families who just get together to eat; we should be families who get together to move and have fun. My mother is seventy-two years young and she still goes dancing two nights a week. I am definitely my mama's daughter. I have always loved to go out dancing, but hold up—I'm no Beyoncé.

Growing up, we would go out roller-skating on Saturday nights and be up on Sunday mornings for church. From swimming to gymnastics to track and field to softball to cheerleading, I've always been involved in sports, and I am determined to leave a legacy of wholeness in health for people to live a more purposeful and meaningful life. I want my grandchildren to grow up with a desire to be healthy mentally, spiritually, and physically.

When I talk to people around this world, they all share the same story: they want better lives for their children than what they had growing up. So when someone comes up to me 50 pounds overweight and says, "I don't have time to work out or cook healthy food. I have to work, and I have family responsibilities," my response is "But don't you want to set a good example for your children? Don't you want a better life for them?" We may not want to improve our health for ourselves, but we'll do anything for our kids.

Just ask Pete Trevino, who lost 30 pounds last year and ran his first half marathon after having one of those aha moments. "I was playing with my two kids, chasing them up the stairs, and when I got to the top, I was totally out of breath," Pete recounted. "I thought, 'I am only thirty years old. I should not be this winded.'" At that moment, Pete decided it was time to stop making excuses and

---

SWEET TWEET

U are a light, so make sure U shine bright. Souls are hungry so get it right!

Share your faith & lift it high. God is not far but nigh!

start taking action. He began my fitness program, dropped 30 pounds, and discovered a whole new way of life.

Pete admits that before he began to care for his health, he made frequent trips to fast-food restaurants and rarely worked out. "My little girl, who is two and a half, could spot those golden arches a mile away, and she'd start asking for chicken nuggets," he said. "I knew it wasn't right to tell her she couldn't have fast food while Daddy was eating it on a regular basis." So the Trevino family made some changes. They began cooking healthy food and walking together as a family. After figuring out a 1.1 mile course, Pete, his wife, and his two children started making that trek several times a week. "My kids are young and they are like little sponges, soaking up everything I do and say. Well, I've been using workout DVDs for some time now, and I caught my six-year-old stepson doing some of the moves from one of the DVDs the other day. I thought that was really cool. My good habits are rubbing off on him."

Pete's story is one we can all relate to. It's never too late to make positive changes that will impact your life and the lives of those you love. Pete would be the first to tell you that it's not always an easy road. In fact, he has lost 30 pounds twice on the way to his goal weight. After losing the first 30 of his 50-pound goal, he regressed and fell back into old eating habits, but he didn't let that deter him. He got right back on the program and has been on track ever since. When he is tempted to fall off the wagon again or when a workout becomes really difficult, Pete just thinks of why he is making the journey in the first place. "I push through the pain and let it remind me that I never want to go back to where I started," he said. "I want to keep setting a good example for my kids."

What better gift can we give our children than the gift of health? Teaching them healthy habits and leading by example is truly living and giving. Proverbs 22:6 says, "Train up a child in the way he should go, and when he is old he will not depart from it." Part of that training should be in the physical realm, and that begins at home.

But you may say, "Donna, I don't know what to do." Well, here are five things you can do to improve the health and well-being of your children and those in your community:

1. ONCE A WEEK, SCHEDULE FAMILY DATE NIGHT. It's a time for the family to move and have fun. Make a list combining each of the family members' favorite activities. Each week choose an activity for family date night, and make it happen.

2. GROW GREEN! Start a family garden, a Garden of Hope (see pages 48–49), or join a community garden. Your family will learn and benefit from growing, cooking, and eating fresh fruits and vegetables. If you are growing your garden indoors and want to give it some pizzazz, the kids can decorate old sneakers and use them as planters. Grown-ups can use old shoes too and create their own personalized planters.

3. PLAN MORE FAMILY MEALS EATEN TOGETHER AT HOME. Use this quality time to talk, share, and learn. Also, get your kids involved in sports and physical activities at schools, community centers, or church.

4. HEART TO HEART: Every month encourage your family to volunteer to help those who are less fortunate. This kind gesture will build character and teach your children to be more humble and giving.

5. EDUCATION: Educate your children about where they come from and their heritage.

Educate your kids to excel in school. As early as first grade, hire a tutor or find a college student who is a volunteer tutor. Adopt the mind-set that your child should excel in every school subject. Don't wait for them to fail. Get them to excel. Educate your children and yourself about the world. Study and learn about other people, cultures, and places. Obtain passports for your entire family. When the opportunity presents itself, travel the world and explore the possibilities of a limitless life. Also, have your child learn another language. We live in a global society, and in order for our children to compete, exceed, and lead in the future, they will need to think of education not as a luxury but as a necessity.

Move to Live

Over years of working in the health and fitness industry, I have discovered that I have to live it to give it. I can't just tell you that movement is important and instruct you to be physically active most days of the week if I am not living it myself. I promise you that I am living it and loving it. I am so passionate about getting you to move, live, and love, because I know these three actions will propel you forward into the life you've always desired. I am in this because I feel called to serve you at a higher level and to make a significant difference. God placed in my heart "move to live, move to give," and I want to pass these words on to you.

The fundamental principal of "move to live, move to give" inspired me to launch the Wobble, Wobble Before You Gobble, Gobble campaign, which began on Thanksgiving Day in 2011. I challenged people to get up and move before eating turkey with all the fixin's and throughout the holiday

> ## BONNAMITE SOUND BITE
>
> Stop making excuses; make a difference instead! Cuz you're not the tail—no way! You're the head!

season. After all, the holiday season is our fattest time of the year. I believe Wobble, Wobble Before You Gobble, Gobble is a wake-up call for America to start a new holiday tradition.

We kicked off the campaign in Miami as part of the city's annual Turkey Trot tradition. The event sold out, with a record 4,500 runners and walkers, including more than 350 children between the ages of two and nine who took part in the Chobani Champions Kids' Trot. It was amazing to spend the morning with so many enthusiastic people. As a group, we gave thanks that we were able to move and participate in such an event, and then I asked everyone to give back not only during the holidays but throughout the year. It was an atmosphere of moving, living, and giving and, boy, was I excited. I was fired up and so was everyone else.

As I walked alongside a father and his daughter, he told me they were spending some special father–daughter time together while Mom was at home cooking. I congratulated him for setting a positive example of good health for his daughter. Next, I met a man who said he had been "forced" to participate in the event by some of his coworkers. "I'm glad to know this Turkey Trot has room for butterballs like me," he joked. "You know what,

Mr. Butterball?" I teased. "I am glad you're here. This is the first step on your road to good health."

As folks crossed the finish line we high-fived each other and celebrated being alive. We also took time to thank the troops by passing out 500 turkeys to military families. It was a great day, and the Wobble, Wobble Before You Gobble, Gobble tradition continues today. In fact, U.S. Surgeon General Dr. Regina M. Benjamin and Cornell McClellan, fellow President's Council member and personal trainer to President and Mrs. Obama, joined me at a kickoff event in Chicago involving the Boys and Girls Clubs of America, where we did the wobble line dance together and encouraged children to make moving and giving a part of their everyday lives. It has become a national call to action—a call to move to live and move to give.

But it all began as a gem of an idea. I knew it wasn't just a good idea; I felt it was a God idea, so I moved on it. I want you to do the same. I want you to get in touch with your higher source and walk in your calling. I want you to wake up every day with the attitude, "This is much bigger than me. I can make a difference in the lives of the people I cross paths with every day."

What Will You Do That Is Significant in the World?

We are in a crisis state today. People are overweight and unhealthy. How can we change the world if we can't even change ourselves? Part of living healthy and whole is realizing that you are a part of something much bigger than you. Make an investment in your health and let it overflow into your families, friends, community, and beyond.

Anyone who is around me very much knows I love sports. I especially love the stories of courage and triumph that often play out in the sports world. One such story that touched my heart, and the hearts of millions around the world, was featured in the 2009 blockbuster film *The Blind Side*. It's the story of Michael Oher, one of his birth mother's thirteen children, who grew up in a tough section of Memphis, Tennessee. He was passed from one foster home to another and eventually found himself homeless and hopeless. On a cold, snowy night in Memphis, with Oher clad in the only clothes he had at the time—a T-shirt and shorts—Leigh Anne Tuohy and her husband, Sean, passed by him in their nice, warm vehicle. She told Sean to turn the car around, and the affluent couple picked up Oher. They immediately fell in love with the six-foot-six, 320-pound sixteen-year-old boy from a bad part of town. Leigh Anne said in an ABC interview, "Michael was there, he had a need, and we had the ability to fill it. . . . He was an instant part of this family."

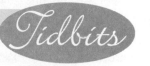

TRANSFORMATION *Tidbits*

- It's never too late to make positive changes that will impact your life and the lives of those you love.

- It's not about your plan but about God's plan for your life.

- Aside from instilling healthy habits in your children, share the gift of giving.

- I want you to wake up every day with the attitude, "This is much bigger than me. I can make a difference in the lives of people I cross paths with every day."

- Move to live, move to give!

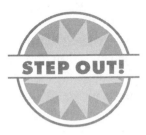

Gandhi once said, "My life is my message." If that's true, what message are you communicating every day? Take a few minutes and jot down three things you'd like to say to the world about the way you live your life.

Sean and Leigh Anne, who already had a daughter and a son at home, helped Oher turn his life around and eventually became Oher's legal guardians when he was seventeen. Leigh Anne made sure he did well in school and on the football field. During his junior year in high school, Oher excelled in football, and by the end of his senior year, he had earned a spot as the starting left tackle on the varsity team. Oher gained a lot of attention for his obvious talent, and many Division I colleges offered him scholarships. In the end, Oher played for the University of Mississippi for four years, and went on to play for the Baltimore Ravens of the NFL. Oher said in an ESPN interview, "I just felt like I was unstoppable. . . . I felt like no matter what, I was going to win the battle."

The Tuohys gave him the unconditional love and encouragement that fueled him on to greatness. The real miracle of the story isn't so much that Oher was discovered and made a name for himself in the NFL—that's just a small part of the picture. The part that touches me so deeply is that Leigh Anne saw a need, had the means to do something about it, and acted on it. She and Sean could've just driven right by that sixteen-year-old boy wearing shorts and a T-shirt on that cold Memphis night, but they didn't. They truly put into action the phrase "move to give."

In an interview following the release of the movie, Leigh Anne said, "My challenge to people is, turn around. Look to your left. Look to your right. That quickly, there can be somebody under

your nose that needs your help and even the smallest bit of kindness—not necessarily bringing them into your home and adopting them, but you know, give a coat to a shelter, and take it [there] yourself. You will get immense satisfaction out of seeing what it does for someone else."

I love the story of moving to give and acting on an opportunity to make a difference in somebody's life. There are many stories of people instilling hope in others. We need to celebrate those people and emulate them. When I think of someone who truly moves to give, I think of one of my heroes: Oprah Winfrey. Anyone who has watched her TV show during the past two and half decades knows that she is a teacher. She has taught me and millions around the world to better ourselves and live more meaningful lives. She has inspired us and challenged us to share our talents and give to others. I've marveled at her willingness to take part in a plethora of philanthropic ventures.

One of her greatest assignments is the Oprah Winfrey Leadership Academy for Girls in South Africa. Having grown up in an impoverished household herself, Oprah always expresses how thankful she is for her education—an education that gave her the foundation to accomplish all the amazing things she's achieved in her lifetime. Oprah wanted to give young girls from poverty-stricken communities the opportunity of a quality education. She believes that "when you teach a girl, you teach a nation." In January 2007 she opened the Academy, fulfilling the promise she had made to former president Nelson Mandela. She built a state-of-the-art facility and instills greatness in these girls, so maybe they can become leaders who will change and impact the world. I am honored and humbled to have worked for several years with her amazing and ambitious girls, teaching them the importance of a healthy mind, spirit, and body.

I was honored to be present for the first graduating class from Oprah's school; seventy-two poised and purposeful young women walked across that stage and accepted their well-deserved diplomas. Now they are in college and pursuing their dreams. Ma Oprah's voice clearly resonates: "There is no bar." I repeat her words: There is no bar. All things are possible! Oprah is the pinnacle example of "move to give." Contribute your time, energy, and resources to helping others. This, by and large, will impact generations to come.

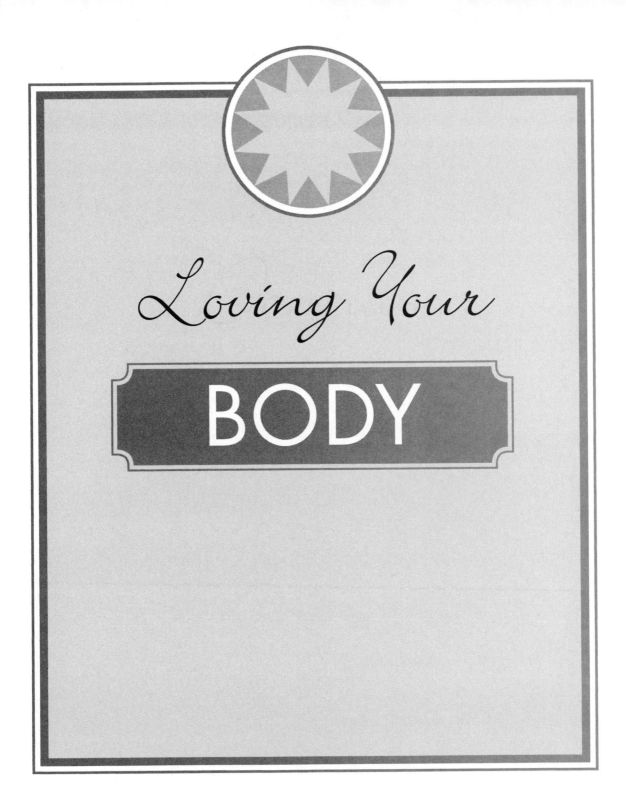

Loving Your

BODY

Eat to Live

As I grew up in church, food was a big part of my life. When I think about those days, I can tell you who made the best pies and cakes for the bake sales. I even remember who made the best food for our church picnics. My life was centered around food—at family reunions, baptisms, weddings, funerals, birthdays, graduations, and other gatherings.

Unfortunately, some of this delicious food was unhealthy. There is absolutely nothing wrong with praying for good health, but there is something wrong with praying for good health while indulging yourself with fried pork chops, fried potatoes, fried chicken, and fried okra. (I'm sure you get the picture.)

Some of you may feel burdened by your bottomless appetites and stuck in an unhealthy lifestyle, but there is hope for you today. Food isn't about wearing shackles; it's about freedom. You have the freedom to choose the foods that are delicious, enjoyable, and life sustaining for your body, soul, and spirit.

That's what Oscar winner Jennifer Hudson did. She went from a size 16 to a size 6, shedding more than 80 pounds on her highly publicized weight-loss journey. The actress-singer said she had to break her "diet mentality" to lose the weight and maintain her new sleek physique. In an interview in *Self* magazine, she said, "I used to deprive myself, thinking that was healthy. I didn't eat pasta, fried food, or red meat. I hadn't had pizza in ten years. . . . If you're on a strict diet that says you shouldn't have any carbs or this or that, your body won't function the way it should. I know now that I can eat anything I want and still lose or maintain my weight. It's about portions and balance."

Hudson lost 60 pounds in 2004 but had gone about it the wrong way, eating only skinless chicken breast, brown rice, and veggies and working out twice a day. She couldn't maintain the weight loss back then because her strict diet and workout rou-

---

SWEET TWEET

U may be tempted at times 2 bend but U won't break. RISE, SHINE, become awake!

Your spirit will change the environment. 2 hope, U are God-sent!

BONNAMITE SOUND BITE

Don't be eatin' that junk that goes straight to your trunk. Know when to say enough is enough! Eat the right way and you'll be struttin' your stuff!

tine weren't realistic. "What are you going to do once you lose weight? Eat everything you gave up!" she explained. Hudson said that once she started following a nutritious, varied diet plan and working out but not overdoing it, she achieved her goal weight and has maintained it ever since.

What about you? What is your attitude toward food? Do you eat to live or live to eat? Do you eat to comfort yourself when you're feeling down or anxious or insecure? Do you reward yourself by eating when you get a promotion at work or finally balance the checkbook? We're all guilty of occasionally eating for the wrong reasons, but if it becomes a way of life, it can lead to an unhealthy relationship with food. The key is to look at food from a different point of view—not as a crutch or a reward, but as something that nourishes you.

First Corinthians 6:19–20 says, "Do you not know that your bodies are temples of the Holy Spirit, who is in you, whom you have received from God? You are not your own; you were bought at a price. Therefore honor God with your bodies." Open up your heart to God's guidance toward a healthy lifestyle, healthy eating, and longevity. Take care of your temple! With God's grace, ask

yourself the following questions: Am I ready to feed and nurture my body and soul? Am I ready to take the steps to honor my temple? If you answered yes, let's get started!

My 28 Days journey will transform your health and your life. With regular workouts, good nutrition, and daily prayer, you will lose weight, feel better, and gain confidence while strengthening your relationship with God. Keep in mind that I am here for you every step of the way. I am here to inspire, serve, and pray for you.

The Right Fuel

We're always putting fuel in our bodies, but we need to feed ourselves the *right* fuel. Don't be a fool when it comes to your fuel! We get more energy from natural foods than we do from processed or packaged foods. Eating natural foods—foods with few or no additives—helps our bodies operate at a much higher level, but those foods aren't always readily available. I found this out the hard way when I was leading my fitness program at an all-girls college in Greensboro, North Carolina. I got the students fired up about working out and eating healthy, and then we went into the college cafeteria, and there weren't any fresh vegetables or fruit. All the meats were swimming in sauces or fried beyond recognition. Plus, many of the dishes were sugary; the students might enjoy the sugar high right after a meal, but later they would crash and burn, making it hard to learn.

I looked at our eating options and thought, "Oh Lord, we have some work to do." So that's what we did—we went to work and planted a garden on the college campus. The Garden of Hope still exists today and provides fresh produce and organic options for the students, faculty, and community.

That experience prompted me to create a program that teaches both children and adults how to grow fresh produce and include it in healthy meals. Grow Green Get Fit gives children as well as their parents gardening tips and teaches them to be healthy physically, nutritionally, and environmentally. It is a twelve-week curriculum being taught at YMCAs, churches, and schools around the country.

Aside from Grow Green Get Fit, I am honored and humbled to be an ambassador for First Lady Michelle Obama's Let's Move initiative, which focuses on creating a healthy start for children, empowering parents and caregivers, providing healthy food in schools, improving access to healthy, affordable foods, and increasing physical activity. I was so excited to help kick off the Let's Move Faith and Communities initiative to help churches and organizations around the country lead healthier and more active lifestyles.

Thanks to Michelle Obama and President Obama for inspiring me to start another program, Gardens of Hope. It is helping people establish gardens of hope to nourish their bodies and souls. It started at home with my dad and my best friend Pat and her son E. J., planting their own gardens and sharing their harvests with their loved ones. And it started with my extended family, the Boys and Girls Clubs of America, and being able to share with them for the past twenty years programs ranging from sports to nutrition.

We have to get serious about the health of children today. I serve on the advisory board of the Robert Wood Johnson Foundation, where our goal is to stop childhood obesity by 2015. According to the Alliance for a Healthier Generation, in the United States one in three children between the ages of two and nineteen are already overweight or obese, and overweight kids are more likely to become overweight adults. Some experts believe that if obesity in our children continues at this rate, our current generation could become the very first in U.S. history to live shorter lives than their parents. When I was growing up there were maybe a handful of overweight kids in every class at school.

Healthy, Hunger-Free Kids Act: Making a Difference in Today's Schools

On December 13, 2010, President Obama signed the Healthy, Hunger-Free Kids Act, which reauthorized the Child Nutrition Act. The House of Representatives had passed the bill on December 2, following a unanimous Senate vote in the summer. According to the Healthy Schools Campaign (HSC) website, the bill includes health-promoting school food policies, such as setting improved commonsense nutrition standards for all school meals and making sure that healthy-living messages are consistent throughout a school's vending machines, stores, and more.

HSC's president and CEO, Rochelle Davis, said this bill was good news for children's health: "In a time when far too many children face both hunger and obesity, this bill presents an opportunity to set policy that will bring healthier food to the children who need it most. . . . We will continue working with hardworking and creative school food-service leaders to support their efforts to bring the healthiest meals possible to students."

They stood out because they were "the fat kids." Today when I go to schools and speak to children, I'm hard-pressed to find a handful of fit kids in every class. Fat has become the new norm and that is scary. That's why I am such an advocate of getting our children moving their bodies and eating healthy. But they can't eat the right fuel if they don't have access to fresh fruits and vegetables. We must do better, for our children and for ourselves.

Yes, I know fresh or organic fruits and vegetables can be a little pricey at the grocery store, so if you are able, buy fresh produce at farmers' markets or grow your own. Take the example of the Garden of Hope, and make an investment in your health and the health of your family. Stop filling your body with chemical-laden foods, which weigh you down and make you feel sluggish. Your body is not designed to process these chemicals. It's just like when you try to save a few bucks and put a low-grade fuel in your car—it doesn't run as smoothly as when you fuel it with the recommended premium grade, right? You'll be sitting at a stoplight and your car is putt-putting, jerking something awful and emitting foul smells, and you're saying, "That ain't me!" It's embarrassing! After an experience like that, you promise to do better, and the next time you pull into a gas station you put the good stuff in your tank. Well, why should you do any less for your body? With the right fuel, you'll rule!

This program is all about putting good fuel into

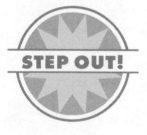

STEP OUT!

In this chapter, we talked about the importance of eating mostly whole foods, but if you are going to buy any packaged food items, you need to know how to read their Nutrition Facts labels. As with anything else, practice makes perfect. Besides telling you the calories per serving, the label shows you both the good stuff—fiber, potassium, vitamins, and minerals—and the bad—sodium, cholesterol, and fat (both saturated and trans fats)—and it includes a list of the ingredients.

Say you're looking for the best cereal to eat. Two different brands may have the same amount of calories but one could be higher in trans or saturated fats, sodium, or sugar. The best foods are low in all three. The ingredients may say plain old sugar, but look for other sweeteners too, such as high-fructose corn syrup. The less sweetener, the better. The ingredients list will also tell you the amount of whole grains included. For example, whole-wheat flour is better than wheat flour because it's made with whole grains instead of processed grains, and it has more fiber.

In general, the fewer the ingredients, the better. Products with a long list of ingredients often contain chemicals and preservatives. Good old Quaker Oats has only one ingredient: "100% Natural Whole Grain Quaker Quality Rolled Oats"!

Here's your assignment. Practice comparing packaged food items. Study their nutritional facts, so you can figure out which would be better for you.

your body and transforming your daily habits, your food choices, and your overall life. When you eat better, your body responds positively and you feel better.

The Winning Formula

My Feed Your Body, Feed Your Soul program will teach you about healthy food choices, portion control, and balance. In fact, you will notice almost immediately how motivated you feel to drop those pounds. Together, we are going to minimize caffeine and reduce processed foods, sugary sodas, and refined sugars, replacing them with delicious meals and snacks that'll keep you energized throughout the day.

The basic equation for weight loss is that the energy in (calories eaten) must be less than the energy out (calories burned). By reducing your calorie intake with this meal plan, increasing your energy with workouts, and showing God gratitude for the strength he provides us, you *will* lose weight.

Ready for the next step? The meal plan is your key to successful eating and weight loss. It's great for both women and men, regardless of your lifestyle, and will maximize your ability to melt away fat and build lean muscle. All the meals contain approximately 40 percent carbohydrate, 30 percent protein, and 30 percent fat. These are meals with maximum nutritional value that will keep you inspired and at your peak performance level.

This amazing plan is designed for you to follow for the next 28 days, or longer if you choose. Each day provides approximately 1,400 calories, which includes breakfast, lunch, dinner, and snacks. Craving variety? Feel free to swap the meals—a breakfast for a breakfast, a lunch for a lunch, and so on. It's as flexible as you need it to be, because all your meals have a low glycemic load with a combination of good carbohydrates, lean proteins, low saturated fats, and limited added sugar. So you have many options and lots of diversity. And most important, you'll feel satisfied and happy!

Especially in the beginning, 1,400 calories may be too low for you. No problem! This plan can be increased to 1,600, 1,800, or 2,000 calories. Just select additional snacks from the snack lists provided on page 53 (the 100-calorie snack list or the 200-calorie snack list). I recommend that you incorporate the additional snacks between meals. And don't forget: always drink a minimum of eight glasses of water a day, or more if you're exercising, to keep your body hydrated.

To formulate your caloric intake, multiply your current weight by ten. Then choose the calorie level closest to your results: 1,400, 1,600, 1,800, or 2,000. This will be a calorie level that should produce weight loss in most individuals. Make sure you never go below 1,400 calories or above 2,000 calories per day.

Don't forget: food is fuel. It's God's gift to us. It keeps us able to function and thrive. Learning the basics about food will be your key to great workouts and successful weight loss, and smart food choices will lead to a healthier you.

Here's the scoop on carbohydrates, proteins, and fats. Not all carbohydrates are created equal. In fact, healthy carbs play a key role in any well-balanced nutrition program. And when chosen correctly, carbs can provide long-lasting energy. But like anything else, it comes down to making the right choices. Learn from the nutritional program to pick nutrient-dense carbohydrates with a low glycemic index, such as fruits, veggies, whole grains, and even moderate amounts of dairy. These healthy carbs can benefit the body. Just be careful: even though healthy carbs aren't fattening, too much of anything can slow your progress, and we don't want that.

Now let's talk about the not-so-healthy carbs, also known as refined carbs and sugar. You'll find them in foods like white bread, sugary sodas, and candy. These unhealthy carbs provide empty calories and have a high glycemic index, meaning they'll give you an immediate spike in energy followed by a rapid plunge, which leaves you tired and sluggish. And who wants to feel like that? So if you need a pick-me-up, go for the healthy fruit or yummy veggies with a little lean protein instead.

Whether it's part of a meal or a snack, protein is essential for life. It feeds your muscles, and this is crucial to your body's reshaping. A healthy balanced diet with plenty of protein will allow your muscles to grow and replace fat tissue with firmness. So eating protein is a win-win. Some great lean protein choices include eggs and egg whites, skinless white-meat poultry, low-fat dairy, and fish. You'll find all these healthy options in abundance throughout the nutrition program in this book. Power up with protein!

We live in a society where fatty foods are plentiful, but as with carbohydrates, there are good fats and bad fats. Good fats, with omega-3 and omega-6 fatty acids, are essential to a well-balanced diet. Some of my favorites throughout this meal plan include olive oil, nuts, and avocados. Healthy fat helps stabilize blood sugar, supply energy, and control hunger. To help you care for your temple, we've taken the liberty of limiting almost all bad fats in the meal plan.

The Witness to Fitness meal plan is about looking and feeling your best. It's also about being spiritually fit and having wholeness in your life. The foundation of the program is the glycemic index—how your blood sugar reacts to the foods you eat. Many fruits, vegetables, lean proteins, and whole grains have a low glycemic index and will provide energy to sustain you throughout your day. To really maximize your stamina, we've taken this one step further, combining foods that have a low glycemic load with a careful balance of proteins, carbs, and fats, to promote optimal control of your blood sugar levels and support your workouts.

On the flip side, I'll repeat: while white bread, sugary sodas, and candy might be your favorites, they simply aren't good for you. After you choose healthy foods over sugary treats for several weeks, you'll kick the junk-food habit and be well on your way to a strong, healthy body.

Even though the Witness to Fitness 28 Days meal plan includes plenty of snacks to satisfy your hunger cravings, I wanted to give you even more options between meals. These snacks are 100 to 200 calories each, yet they are filling and will help keep your hunger to a minimum throughout the day. Be sure you mix it up when choosing healthy snacks, so you won't become bored and reach for a calorie-laden treat.

The following snacks may be used to increase your daily caloric intake in case the original 1,400-calorie meal plan is not enough for your current starting weight.

TRANSFORMATION *Tidbits*

- When you eat better, your body responds positively and you feel better.
- Get into the habit of planning your meals for the entire week.
- When you go out to eat, ask yourself, "Will this meal treasure or trash my temple?"
- When you power up with healthy food, fitness, and faith, you power up every aspect of your life.

100-CALORIE SNACKS

- 1 ounce skinless white-meat chicken breast with 1 ounce low-fat Swiss cheese and 3 whole-wheat crackers
- 1 ounce ham with 1 ounce low-fat cheddar cheese and 3 whole-wheat crackers
- 1 ounce sliced white-meat turkey with ¼ avocado and 1 rice cake
- ½ apple with 2 teaspoons all-natural peanut butter
- ½ apple with 3 tablespoons hummus
- 1 skim-milk mozzarella string cheese stick with ½ cup cantaloupe
- 2 slices tomato with 1 ounce skim-milk mozzarella cheese, plus vinegar, salt, and pepper to taste
- ½ cup blueberries, ¼ cup low-fat cottage cheese, and 3 almonds

200-CALORIE SNACKS

- 2 ounces sliced white-meat turkey, 1 ounce reduced-fat Swiss cheese, and 10 grapes
- 2 hard-boiled eggs and ½ cup cantaloupe
- 1 8-inch celery stalk and 8 baby carrots with tuna salad (3 ounces white-meat tuna mixed with 1 tablespoon light mayonnaise)
- 1 ounce roast beef rolled with ½ apple, sliced, and 1 slice reduced-fat Swiss cheese
- 2 ounces ham with 1 ounce low-fat cheddar cheese and 4 whole-wheat crackers
- 1 apple with 1 tablespoon all-natural peanut or almond butter
- 8 baked tortilla chips with ¼ cup hummus, celery sticks, and red bell pepper slices
- 1 toasted whole-wheat English muffin topped with 1 ounce sliced white-meat turkey, ½ ounce reduced-fat Swiss cheese, and 1 slice tomato

Just Say No

Now let's talk about what you won't be eating. You know, balanced eating doesn't mean holding a cookie in each hand. Simply put, you should limit the amount of "man's creations" in your daily meal plan. These are the foods you generally find on the inner aisles of a supermarket, the items that come in boxes and bags. Not all the foods lining the inner aisles of a grocery store are bad for you; some we'll call "neutral." And others, such as canned beans and frozen vegetables or fruit, offer a convenient way to eat healthy foods. Many of them, however, trigger cravings, hunger, and fat storage. They're high in calories but low in nutritional value. It's especially important to limit the following:

- Soda, fruit drinks, sports drinks, or other sugar-added beverages
- White foods: white flour, white bread, white rice, and white pasta
- Processed snack foods, such as potato chips, cheese puffs, and pork rinds
- Sweets—candy, cookies, cake, etc.
- Foods high in sugar, high-fructose corn syrup, or molasses
- Fried foods

- Caffeine

- Fatty meats, such as bacon and sausage

- Foods that are high in sodium (Watch out for frozen dinners and canned soups.)

- Most fast food (Some chains offer healthier options, so if you have to choose fast food, stick with those.)

- Alcohol (These calories add up, especially since alcohol is usually consumed at night when you're less likely to burn calories. Alcohol may also increase hunger, making it harder to resist tempting treats that you'll regret later.)

If you're used to eating fatty, fried foods or living off food that is handed to you from a drive-through window, you may feel deprived when you start limiting yourself. Eventually, though, your taste will adjust and you won't crave the unhealthy choices so much. Also, as the pounds start to drop, it will inspire you to keep eating right.

Success Strategies

There's more to winning a battle of the bulge than simply knowing what to eat and what to avoid. To accomplish anything important in life, you need a good strategy—whether it's getting a job, studying for a test, hunting for a house, or raising a child. Why would losing weight be any different? Here are some success strategies that will help you develop better eating habits and aid you in your weight-loss program:

- Eat slowly and take small bites. This helps you better appreciate what you're eating. Plus, it's good for your digestion.

- Put down the fork and try eating with chopsticks. You will end up taking smaller bites.

- Eat meals at the table. Avoid eating while watching TV, walking down the street, or driving in your car. If you're distracted, you're more likely to overeat.

- If you're still hungry after eating a snack or a meal, wait twenty minutes before eating more, because it takes that long for your system to register that you are full.

- Keep healthy snacks in your bag. An apple or a small bag of almonds can satisfy any hunger pangs during the day.

- Avoid eating late, because you're less likely to burn off the calories thereafter. If you're starving, have a light snack, preferably fruit or vegetables.

- Eat an apple before lunch or dinner. This will make you less likely to overindulge.

- Drink plenty of water. It may satisfy your craving.

These strategies might feel odd at first, especially if you're used to eating dinner in three minutes flat while watching your favorite TV show or wolfing down a burger and fries while driving home from work. However, if you keep practicing these strategies, eventually they'll turn into habits.

Here are my top success strategies for eating out without gaining weight:

- Split in two—it's the right thing to do! Ask the waiter in advance to divide your meal into two equal servings, serve you only half and give you the remaining half in a doggie bag. That way, you are guaranteed not to eat it all at one time.

- Bye-bye bread. If you allow yourself to have bread with your meal, take one small piece then ask the waiter to remove the bread basket from your table. You won't have to eye it, and it won't have to eye you.

- Drink up! And I mean H_2O. The only time it's okay to drink and drive is when you're downing a bottle of water on your way to a restaurant. Ask the waiter to keep the water flowing at the table. Drinking plenty of water fills up your stomach, so you won't overeat at the restaurant. It's a win-win.

- Sweetened drinks are loaded with calories, so just stick to plain old water. You're probably saying, "Donna, you are a party pooper!" But hey, I'm just trying to be a role model. Remember this: take in less, fit in the dress.

- Restaurant desserts are also loaded with calories, so share it, don't wear it! Or simply look for bite-size portions. It will save you money and put less weight on you, honey!

Restaurants are great at creating menus that have delicious-sounding appetizers and entrées. Many times these meals sound fairly healthy but are really very high in fat and calories. Use the tips below to help you interpret the menu items at your favorite restaurant:

- Order protein that is described as "grilled," "broiled," "poached," or "wood-fired." Use caution with anything described as "breaded," "crispy," or "fried."

- Ask for sauces and dressings on the side, or request a low-calorie alternative red- or white-wine sauce. Any sauce described as "creamy" or "buttery" will be very high in fat and calories.

- Ask for steamed vegetables instead of heavy starches, such as french fries or baked potatoes.

The good news about fast-food and chain restaurants is that they usually have nutritional information available on their websites and menus. I encourage you to check out the calorie count of the appetizers and entrées you enjoy. In my meal plan, we aim for a breakfast of 300 calories and lunches and dinners of 400 calories each. You can use the nutritional information listed for all the meals and snacks in this guide as a rule of thumb when ordering from menus that contain nutritional information.

I know that on occasion, fast-food and chain restaurants are convenient. Life gets too hectic to cook and prepare all your meals all the time. And while home-cooked food is always best, going out is sometimes the only option. Some eating-out

Smart Eating

The key to controlling your weight and improving your health is to practice good nutrition. Read your food labels and check over the nutritional facts to ensure that you are eating foods high in nutritional value.

tips will help you navigate the world of menus and drive-through. Below are the biggest mistakes that people make while eating out:

- THE BREAD BASKET: An average dinner roll can have anywhere from 100 to 200 calories, and that's before you add any butter. Do yourself a favor and ask the server to remove the bread from your table.

- DESSERT: If you are craving something sweet after dinner, wait until you get home, where you know the calories of the foods you are eating. Restaurant desserts are often loaded with calories, but look for bite-size desserts.

Mealtime Makeover

One habit you don't want to develop is skipping meals. If you get busy during the day it can be tempting to skip meals, but that is a bad idea! When you skip meals, your metabolism slows down in order to conserve energy. And when your metabolism slows down, you burn fewer calories and become more sluggish. Skipping a meal also makes you more likely to overeat at the next meal. This is particularly bad if you're skipping lunch, because you'll overeat at dinner and have less time to burn off the additional calories. Some health experts advocate eating five or six small meals instead of three larger meals, which keeps your metabolism revved up all day long. The bottom line is, weight loss does not mean starvation.

Sometimes people skip meals simply because they haven't planned ahead. Eating healthy and losing weight is so much easier if you do a little prep work. The extra planning takes a little time but makes a huge difference. Get into the habit of planning your meals for an entire week. Do your major food shopping over the weekend and begin cooking your meals for the week ahead. Get creative! Use the recipes from the meal plan in the 28 Days program, consult healthy cookbooks, read healthy-living magazines, ask friends for their favorite healthy recipes, and search the Internet for ideas.

Even if you don't have time to prepare your meals a week in advance, make sure you stock your fridge and cabinets with healthy foods so there's always something you can grab on the go. If you have good food in the house, you'll be less likely to stop for fast food or order takeout when it's time to eat. Even if you choose seemingly healthy options, like salad or soup, calories can sneak in via salad dressings and cream bases. And you have no idea what the chef is putting in the dish you ordered. You can't control it, but you can control what goes into your culinary creations at home.

When you're cooking, make big portions of healthy dishes and save the leftovers. Soups and stews are perfect for this. You can also make a huge salad and eat it for days. Just make sure to put dressing only on what you plan to eat at each sitting so your leftovers won't be soggy.

This program of healthy eating and exercise will have you looking leaner and feeling your best almost immediately. Once you've completed your 28 days, you can jump back in and repeat the meal plan; swap the breakfasts, lunches, dinners, and snacks for more variety; or turn to the easy-to-use substitution lists on pages 57–59 to further customize the plan.

Don't like an item on the meal plan? Or just looking for a little more variety? Simply select from the substitution lists and customize your plan to your personal lifestyle and taste preferences.

Protein

SWAP THIS	EAT THIS
1 ounce skinless white poultry, such as chicken or turkey breast, or 1 ounce tuna	¾ ounce lean roast beef 1 ounce lean pork chops or pork tenderloin 1 egg or 3 egg whites ¾ ounce salmon or other oily fish 1 ounce shrimp or other lean seafood, such as tilapia or cod
1 egg	3 egg whites 1½ ounces lean skinless white poultry or seafood 1½ ounces lean pork chop or pork tenderloin 1 ounce hamburger or other red meat 1 ounce salmon or other oily fish
1 ounce salmon or other oily fish	1½ ounces tuna or other lean seafood 1½ ounces skinless white poultry 1½ ounces lean pork chop or pork tenderloin ⅓ cup low-fat cottage cheese 1 ounce hamburger or other red meat
1 ounce shrimp or other lean fish, such as tilapia or cod	¾ ounce lean roast beef 1 ounce lean pork chops or pork tenderloin ¼ cup canned string beans, cooked 1 egg or 3 egg whites ¾ ounce salmon or other oily fish 1 ounce skinless white poultry or tuna
1 ounce hamburger or other red meat	1½ ounces skinless white poultry 1½ ounces tuna or other lean seafood 1½ ounces lean pork chop or pork tenderloin 1 ounce salmon or other lean fish 1 egg or 3 egg whites ⅓ cup low-fat cottage cheese

Dairy

SWAP THIS	EAT THIS
1 cup skim milk or low-fat soy milk	½ cup low-fat cottage cheese 1 cup plain nonfat yogurt 1 ounce reduced-fat cheese 1 egg
1 ounce reduced-fat cheese	1 egg 1 cup skim milk or low-fat soy milk ½ cup low-fat cottage cheese 2 ounces lean meat, such as turkey 1 tablespoon peanut butter ½ cup low-fat yogurt
½ cup low-fat cottage cheese	1 cup skim milk or low-fat soy milk ½ cup low-fat yogurt 1 egg or 3 egg whites 1 tablespoon peanut butter 2 ounces lean meat, such as turkey
1 cup low-fat yogurt	1 cup low-fat cottage cheese 2 eggs or 6 egg whites

Fruit

All of the following are equal to a single serving of fruit and are interchangeable:

1 medium apple	2 small plums
15 grapes	15 cherries
1 orange	1 small grapefruit
2 kiwifruits	1 small pear
1 cup melon	1 cup berries
1 peach	½ cup pineapple
½ banana	

Vegetables

All of the following are equal to a single serving of vegetables and are interchangeable:

1 cup broccoli, string beans, spinach, or cauliflower, steamed	1 whole tomato
1 cup raw chopped veggies, such as cucumber, pepper, or celery	12 cherry or grape tomatoes
10 brussels sprouts, steamed	3 cups lettuce
	12 asparagus spears, steamed

Carbohydrates

SWAP THIS	EAT THIS
Half a 6-inch whole-wheat pita pocket	1 slice whole-wheat bread 1 light whole-grain English muffin 1 small whole-grain dinner roll 90 calories worth of whole-grain crackers
½ cup whole-grain pasta or couscous, cooked	⅓ cup brown rice, steamed 1 slice whole-wheat bread 1 small whole-grain dinner roll 1 small baked potato or sweet potato
1 slice whole-wheat bread	1 light whole-grain English muffin 1 small whole-grain dinner roll 90 calories worth of whole-grain crackers Half a 6-inch whole-wheat pita pocket
⅓ cup brown rice, steamed	½ cup whole-grain pasta or couscous, cooked ⅓ cup barley or quinoa, cooked 1 small baked potato or sweet potato 1 slice whole-wheat bread
1 cup steel-cut oatmeal, cooked	1 cup whole-grain cereal 1½ slices whole-wheat bread 1 whole-wheat English muffin 1 cup cream of wheat 1½ whole-grain waffles

Lastly, let's discuss portion size. You may order a very healthy meal but still end up with too many calories. This is because many restaurants serve enormous portions. When your dish arrives at the table, survey the size of the meal. If it looks large, cut it in half and take home a doggie bag. You can also share your meal.

Be your own advocate. Keep in mind that restaurant food can be mysterious. Even the most healthy-sounding menu item can show up with unforeseen heavy sauces. Ask your server what the lighter menu items are. When in doubt, ask for your food to be grilled or broiled, with the sauce on the side.

As you begin to change your eating lifestyle, meditate on 1 Corinthians 10:31, which says, "Whether you eat or drink, or whatever you do, do all to the glory of God." Trust your inner voice. When you go out to eat, ask yourself, "Will this meal treasure or trash my temple?" Take a photo of your meal and keep a food journal. Keep in mind that by making healthier food choices you are taking steps into the newness of a healthier you.

Information in this chapter and in the daily program is from the Body Gospel Nutrition Guide. Please go to Beachbody.com for the complete Body Gospel fitness program and nutrition guide, and for your other health and fitness needs.

8

Move to Live

I have this relative who was obese, yet he wouldn't do anything about it. Every time I saw him, I'd encourage him to move. He'd always look me in the eyes and say, "Now, Donna, I'm gonna start walking." The first nine or ten times he told me that, I smiled sweetly and nodded, but I finally let him know what was on my mind: "If you added up all the times you told me you were going to start walking, you could've walked to California and back by now." He didn't have a response for that because he knew I was right. I told him, if you can move your body, then you are not exempt from working out. I don't want any woulda-shoulda-coulda excuses for not being physically active. Those excuses don't fly with me. Besides, I've heard every excuse in the book, and I have the same response to each one: your body needs movement to be healthy, so get moving!

I used to say, "If people knew better, they'd do better," but I don't say that anymore. The truth is, some people do know better and *still* choose not to do better when it comes to their health. I want you to think of your health as the power line of your life. Power lines provide electricity so things like your toaster, your lamp, your iPod charging station, and your computer will function. Your body is the same way. It won't function unless you power it with good health. And, baby, I'm sure you could use a charge right about now. You have to eat to live, move to live, de-stress to live, have faith to live, and all of those things work together for the sake of your health, which gives energy to your life.

I once saw an advertisement that said, "Exercise. You don't have time not to." Truer words were never spoken. Your attitude toward fitness has to change. You have to conceive it; then you will receive it. Movement has to be a part of your everyday life, if you wish to achieve and maintain a strong, healthy body. So many people moan and groan when they hear the word "exercise." They think it's going to be painful, uncomfortable, and

---

SWEET TWEET

Take a deep breath 2 release your stress.
It's a new day given to U to be blessed.

Move your body from side to
side. Jump, leap, & slide!

horrible. So let's start by giving exercise another name. Let's call it movement or physical activity. Let's think of it as something we were meant to do, because we were. We have to make physical activity a priority. Look at being healthy as a responsibility to energize your being. When you power up with healthy food, fitness, and faith, you power up every aspect of your life.

Here's how I keep the energy flowing in my life. I start my day with prayer and meditation. I speak to God, and I listen to my spirit. Then I work out. If I feel the need to rev up my mojo later, I put on my favorite music and dance and sing with every fiber of my being. Truth be told, I can't sing a lick, but that doesn't stop me from making a joyful noise. You see, it does not matter what activity you do or when you do it; you will feel so much better if you just get moving.

The late great singer James Brown said it like this: "Get up offa that thing and shake till you feel better." I'm echoing his words and saying, "Let's move to improve!" Movement is healthy. Movement is devotion. Movement is joy. Movement is freedom of expression and good for your body and soul. Feel the rhythm of movement and breathe in new life.

Reecie, one of my weight-loss soldiers, had to come to grips with weighing over 400 pounds. She had tried and failed at several other fitness programs before meeting me, but I convinced her that she could succeed this time because she wouldn't be relying on her own strength and willpower; she'd be tapping into her faith. And she is seeing success! As she says, "I'm a work in progress.

"While on my journey," she adds, "Donna challenged me to a half marathon. It changed my life. I never thought that I would have been able to do something like that—me, over 300 pounds at the time. . . . It took me what seemed like forever, but I did it." Reecie said that when she crossed the finish line, she realized she would never have to settle for less again. She knew things were going to be different from that point on in her life. "I didn't have to live with excuses anymore. I can show my children that you can do anything that you put your mind to, and with God's help, it can be done."

Maybe you can relate to Reecie's story. Maybe you need to lose weight, change your ways, or use your passion to push you into your purpose. But you've been making excuses for far too long. Now make better decisions. Well, if you've read this far, good for you! You're taking steps to become

FitnessGram

FitnessGram is a fitness assessment and reporting program for youth, first developed in 1982 by the Cooper Institute in response to the need for a comprehensive set of assessment procedures in physical education programs. The assessment includes a variety of health-related physical fitness tests that assess aerobic capacity, muscular strength, muscular endurance, flexibility, and body composition. Scores from these assessments are compared to Healthy Fitness Zone standards to determine a student's overall physical fitness and suggest areas for improvement when appropriate.

a better you. You're striving for optimum health and abundant life! You've shifted your thinking and found the kind of attitude you need in order to stick to the program. You've looked to your faith for the strength and support to see you all the way through to accomplishing your ultimate goals. You're closer than you think to transforming your mind, spirit, and body.

We've talked in depth about the mental and spiritual components. Now we're ready to focus on the physical. It's time to move to live! We covered proper nutrition and the ways you can incorporate healthy eating into your life in chapter 7. Now let's dive right into the three types of movement you'll need in your fitness program: cardio, strength training, and flexibility.

The Cardio Cure

If you belong to a gym or hang out with fitness-minded people, you're bound to hear the terms "cardio" and "aerobics." "Cardio" is short for cardiovascular exercise, and it is your best friend when trying to lose weight, because cardio burns calories as well as strengthens your heart and lungs. When you hear "aerobics," it might conjure up images of 1980s legwarmers, headbands, and Jane Fonda–type fitness instructors, but the word "aerobic" simply means "with oxygen." The term "aerobics," coined by fitness guru Dr. Kenneth Cooper, refers to up-tempo movement that promotes the circulation of oxygen in the blood. So cardio and aerobics are often interchangeable in conversation and basically mean the same thing: you are going to get your heart rate up, sweat your butt off, and burn some major calories.

Aerobic exercise is different from anaerobic exercise. Aerobics is a continuous activity that you engage in long enough and hard enough to work your heart, lungs, and the large muscle groups (the legs, back, and chest). Conversely, anaerobic exercise is high-intensity movement performed all-out for short periods of time—usually for not more than three minutes—followed by a rest period. Anaerobic exercise involves short bursts of energy, like you might use in sprinting or weightlifting. Jogging around the track for thirty minutes is an aerobic activity, while wind sprints would be considered anaerobic. Both require large muscle groups and both get your heart rate up; however, one is performed for a continuous period of time and the other for short bursts of time.

I play golf and I love what golf teaches you: respect, patience, focus, commitment, and discipline. I serve on the board of the LPGA Foundation and actively work with the Girls Golf program, which gives girls ages seven to seventeen the chance to play golf and build friendships. More than 7,000 girls participate at more than 225 sites around the country. When we work with the girls, we teach them the five Es of Girls Golf: Empower, Enrich, Engage, Exercise, and Energize. These same principles apply to us as we pursue optimum health.

- EMPOWER: Be empowered. You can accomplish anything!

- ENRICH: See the value of health and wellness and recognize that it enriches your life in so many ways.

- ENGAGE: Engage in becoming a witness to fitness.

- EXERCISE: Exercising and becoming more fit increases your self-esteem and will increase your self-confidence.

- ENERGIZE: Energize yourself with enthusiasm for wholeness and newness in your health, and live a more purposeful life.

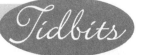

TRANSFORMATION *Tidbits*

- Movement is healthy. Movement is devotion. Movement is joy. Movement is freedom of expression and good for you, body and soul.

- Feel the rhythm of movement and breathe in new life.

- You can break through a plateau and reap the rewards of working out if you incorporate the FITT principle: Frequency, Intensity, Time, and Type.

- Where there's a will, you will find a way.

- Fit in fitness and try my ten-in-ten workout.

- You have to eat to live, move to live, de-stress to live, and have faith to live—all these things work together for the goodness of your health.

Even though golf isn't an aerobic activity, you can make it cardio-friendly by walking the course. Get your butt off the cart and walk instead of ride.

Too often people get locked down into one type of workout. Remember, variety is the key to success. Why not identify physical activities that you enjoy? Do you love riding your bike? Get a bike and hit the trails. Do you love dancing? Take a dance class or simply move to your favorite music and shake your groove thing. Were you the jump-rope king or queen back in the day? Get a jump rope and jump to fitness! Just because you're an adult doesn't mean you can't have fun running, jumping, dancing, and playing around. Just move!

If you are just getting started or haven't been physically active in a while, make sure to check with your doctor before beginning any workout pro-gram. It might be challenging at first, but stay with it. The key is to start at a level you're comfortable with and build from there. In other words, don't try to run a 10K on your first day. Rather, begin by walking fifteen to thirty minutes every day and increase your activity from that point. Need some more motivation to get started? Take it from Pastor Lawrence Robinson, from the Potter's House in Dallas, Texas: working out is worth your time.

In October 2010, Pastor Robinson noticed that his legs were swollen and that he was putting on a little weight. His doctor gave him medicine for the swelling but he also started walking three miles three times a week. He put in his three miles early on Easter Sunday in 2011, but he just didn't feel right. Still, he walked and prayed and confessed, "I am healed. I am healed." The following Sunday, he became winded while holding his grandchild and climbing the stairs at church. He attributed it to his grandchild getting too big to carry, but that wasn't it. After church, while watching a ball game, he told his wife he didn't feel well, and that night, he woke up at 3:30 A.M. feeling like Muhammad Ali was punching him in the chest. He and his wife headed for the hospital. The next day the doctors discovered that three of the arteries in his heart were totally blocked, and he underwent open-heart surgery.

Upon his release from the hospital, he decided he needed to do things differently: "I needed to change my mind-set and come up with a new game plan." And that's exactly what he did. He began making healthier food choices, he started limiting his portion sizes, and he stopped eating late at night. "I felt like I had a second chance at life. I knew God was keeping me here for a reason. Even though it was through my own negligence that I let my temple get in such poor shape, God gave me another chance to finish the purpose he has for me."

Pastor Robinson knew that in order to complete all his assignments, he would have to get healthier, and he knew he wasn't alone in his plight. As he looked around at his coworkers, he noticed that many of them also needed their temples tuned up. So Pastor Robinson reached out to the men and women in his workplace, encouraging them to see their doctors and commit to a healthier lifestyle. About twenty of his coworkers started getting together weekly for health check-ins, which included sharing health tips and a lot of encouragement. He has also become active in educating himself and others about Alzheimer's and dementia and implementing an Alzheimer's program at his church, since the disease has touched his family. I am excited about my dad's participation and improvement since joining the program. Pastor Robinson is not only helping my dad and others, he realizes that he has a lot of work to do. "I've still got time on my clock," he said. "I don't want to hinder God's work because he can't use me in the way he would like to if I am out of shape."

Pastor Robinson's moment of reckoning came after his heart surgery, but he doesn't want others to wait that long to make healthy lifestyle changes. "It all comes down to discipline," he said. "Making fitness part of your day and eating healthy foods has to become [a] priority. And never quit. When you're down, you can only get back up." This is your time to get back up, or possibly get up for the first time. Pastor Robinson had to change his mind-set and change his habits before he could change his life. You'll have to do the same.

> HERE ARE SOME EXAMPLES OF
> CARDIO YOU MIGHT TRY:
> Walking, hiking, jogging, swimming, biking, dancing, rollerblading, jumping rope, doing water aerobics, or working out with fitness DVDs. When trying something new, don't be discouraged; just pace yourself. Do as much as you can each time. Push yourself but listen to your body.

If you get bored with one activity, switch it up to keep things fresh—Pilates one day, salsa dance class the next. Variation is good for your body, since you're using different muscle groups and challenging your body in new ways. Do anything you can to make it more fun. You might want to start a walking club at your workplace or a fitness club at your church. Exercising with a partner or group keeps you motivated and it can be a great boost to your new healthy lifestyle. Think of friends you'd like to spend more time with and set a time to meet for fitness and fellowship. Make special cardio playlists of your favorite music, which will motivate you to finish every workout strong. I believe that great music can lead to better health. Over the last few years, I've put that theory into practice as I've merged exercise and entertainment into workout videos and TV shows. It's so important to make movement enjoyable, and having great music will keep you moving.

DONNAMITE SOUND BITE

Wallow in God's greatness and his goodness too! Cuz we have some work to do! It won't always be easy, but you've got to move. That's the only way you'll ever improve!

In the 28 Days program at the end of this book, I'll guide you with the amount of cardio you should be doing each day. In general, healthy adults should get at least two and a half hours of moderate aerobic activity every week, according to the Department of Health and Human Services. That may seem like a lot, if you've never been an avid exerciser, but you can do it! Author Samuel Johnson once said, "Clear your mind of can't." I say, "Amen, Samuel!"

Get Strong

"Strength is happiness. Strength is itself victory. In weakness and cowardice there is no happiness." Daisaku Ikeda said it, but we're living it! We're getting stronger in every area of our lives—mentally, spiritually, and physically.

To get stronger physically, strength training is a must. If you've never done resistance training before, you'll be surprised at how quickly you can build strength, feel better, and look your best. Aside from toning your muscles and improving your overall appearance, strength training improves balance and coordination, enhances your posture, increases bone density, and prevents osteoporosis. Stronger muscles and bones make you less prone to injury. Strength training also boosts your metabolism: the more muscle mass you have, the more calories you burn while your body is at rest, especially in the hours just after your workout. And here's some good news: you'll lose weight faster than you would just doing cardio alone. So cardio plus weight training is the key to feeling stronger and looking leaner.

My approach to strength training is the same as it is to cardio: if you're new to it, start out slow and build up intensity and repetitions over time. Strength training is done in sets of repetitions, or

reps. Perform a number of reps to equal one set, and rest from thirty seconds to one minute in between each set; your rest time will depend on your fitness level and the type of activity you are doing. As you get stronger, increase the weight of your dumbbells. In my program, the focus is on using lighter weights (3–10 pounds) and performing more reps, but in other programs the weights will vary.

The most efficient kind of strength training is multimuscle. It's the best way to achieve a total body workout. In multimuscle strength training, you perform two different exercises simultaneously, working two muscle groups. For example, you could do a bicep curl while doing a lunge. This helps you build the same amount of strength in half the time.

Weight training should be done on alternate days, to give your muscles time to rest and recover. However, when you are following a specific strength-training program your regimen will vary. As with cardio, feel free to switch up your exercises to keep it interesting and keep you motivated. All sorts of fitness tools will help you vary your workouts, including kettlebells, medicine balls, bars, and resistance bands.

Your attitude toward strength training will change. No, you're not going to get big and bulky. Yes, you're going to get toned, tight, and trim! Yippee!

The 411 on Flexibility

Our muscles get tighter with age, making everyday tasks like reaching for the top shelf more challenging. So it's important to stretch out your muscles to remain as loose as possible. Stretching is incredibly beneficial; it not only prevents injury and improves flexibility, but also calms your spirit and brings

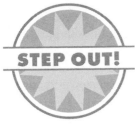

STEP OUT!

To help you move to live, here are my top five favorite smartphone fitness apps to use on your lifelong journey of health and wellness:

1. MyFitnessPal: This free app tracks your food and exercise whenever and wherever you'd like.

2. CalorieKing: This free app gives you quick and easy access to calories, carbs, and fat content of more than 70,000 foods, including meals at 260 fast-food chains and restaurants.

3. Lose It!: This free app helps you set goals and establish a daily calorie budget so you can stay on track every day by recording your food and exercise. More than 85 percent of this app's active users have lost weight.

4. RunKeeper: This free app uses your phone's GPS to track fitness activity, such as how far you run, the amount of time it took you, your pace, speed, calories burned, and much more.

5. AllTrails: A free app for all of you hikers and mountain bikers. It tracks your hikes with your phone's GPS and offers topographic maps, routes, reviews, and driving directions.

peace of mind. Like cardio and strength training, flexibility training is very important to your overall fitness goals. It improves posture and coordination, reduces back pain, increases range of motion, and betters your overall performance in sports.

Before you participate in any physical activity, it's important to warm up. The warm-up prepares your body for activity by elevating your heart rate and increasing blood flow to your muscles. Perform a march or jog for several minutes followed by light stretches that are held for several seconds. The best time to stretch and increase your flexibility is after you work out, which is referred to as your cooldown. The purpose of the cooldown is to lower your heart rate, stretch your muscles to prevent muscle soreness, and reduce your risk of injury. These stretches are held for twenty seconds to one minute. Practice taking deep breaths in and out, and do not bounce when you're stretching.

Think of stretching after your workout as mandatory, not optional . . . you'll feel so much better.

Get FITT

Okay, so you're convinced that you need to incorporate cardio, strength training, and stretching into your everyday life, right? Well, it's more than half the battle just realizing that you need to do these activities and committing to doing them on a regular basis. Now let me go over an important part of fitness training that will help you gauge your workouts and avoid hitting a dreaded plateau.

A plateau occurs when your body does the same activity over and over and becomes proficient at it. When this happens, performing these movements requires less energy and therefore burns fewer calories. But you can break through that plateau and reap the rewards of working out if you incorporate the FITT principle: Frequency, Intensity, Time, and Type. Frequency is how often you exercise. Intensity is the effort you put into it. Time is the length of time devoted to exercising, and Type is the kind of workout. According to the American College of Sports Medicine (ACSM), you should do cardio three to five times a week at an intensity of 60 to 80 percent of your maximum heart rate for twenty to sixty minutes.

To help you work out at the proper level of intensity, you need to know your target heart rate. That formula is the number 220 minus your age multiplied by 60 to 80 percent. Another way of measuring your intensity is through perceived exertion, which is measured by how hard you feel you're working on a scale from one to ten. Ideally, your typical workout should fall between five and eight. Or you can measure your intensity with a talk test. As a general guide, you should be able to carry on a conversation while you are working out. You don't want to be completely out of breath, but your conversation should be breathy.

For strength training, the ACSM recommends working out two to three times a week at an intensity that is 70 to 85 percent of your one-rep maximum (the maximum weight you can lift with good form in one repetition) for eight to ten reps and

one to three sets. Following this suggestion will help you see progressive and positive results.

Fit in Fitness

Again and again I hear the same excuses for not working out, but "I don't have time" consistently tops the list. Although I have addressed the time issue before, I want to repeat that you have to make your health a priority and find ways to fit in fitness. You find time to do all the other things you value. Remember, good health is the power line for your life, so value it!

You can fit in fitness lots of different ways. For example, get your butt up and moving while you're watching TV; during the commercial breaks fit in fitness. Take the stairs instead of the elevator. Park a little farther away and walk to your destination. Dance a little longer on the dance floor. Or walk instead of standing on the moving walkway. Catch my drift? Statistics show that you can burn 300 calories walking up and down stairs for thirty minutes. You can even fit in fitness when you travel. With all of today's travel regulations, you have to arrive at an airport a minimum of one hour before your flight and as much as two to three hours, if you're traveling internationally. Don't sit your butt

BMI

Another fitness formula you'll find helpful is figuring your BMI—body mass index. BMI can be used to indicate if you are overweight, obese, underweight, or normal. To calculate your BMI, use the following formula: BMI = (weight in pounds / [height in inches × height in inches]) × 703. A healthy BMI score is between 20 and 25. A score below 20 indicates that you may be underweight; a value above 25 indicates that you may be overweight.

down and stuff your face; get up and walk the airport like I do. Yes, with my roll-on suitcase and briefcase, I'm walking and burning fat. That's what I call fitness on the move!

Here are my five favorite ways to fit in fitness. Remember, where there's a will, you will find a way!

1. Make it a game: get the family to move with some of the popular fitness and dance games, such as Xbox's "Michael Jackson: The Experience," "Dance Central 2," or "Dance Dance Revolution Universe 3"; Wii's "Dance Dance Revolution Hottest Party 2" or "Dancing with the Stars: We Dance!"; or PlayStation 3's "Everybody Dance" or "The Fight: Lights Out."

2. Sign up for a local 5K or 10K race.

3. Schedule fitness breaks throughout your day:

   Pump up the jam and dance

   Jump rope for ten minutes

   Get your Hula-hoop on

   Stretch at your desk

   Walk for lunch

   Try my ten-in-ten workout with your favorite music—ten moves in ten minutes:

   One minute: jump rope or jump in place

   One minute: walking lunges

   One minute: jumping jacks

   One minute: squats with bounce

   One minute: march or jog in place

   One minute: triceps dips using a chair

   One minute: ski hops from side to side

   One minute: push-ups using a sofa or chair

   One minute: football run turning side to side

   One minute: crunches (as many as possible) on the floor or in a chair

4. Rise and shine: set your alarm clock ten minutes earlier and start your day with a praise and worship dance.

As a member of the President's Council on Fitness, Sports, and Nutrition, I encourage people of all ages, backgrounds, and abilities to get fit and participate in the Presidential Active Lifestyle Award challenge (PALA+). To earn this achievement, adults must perform thirty minutes of physical activity daily, and kids under eighteen must perform sixty minutes of activity daily, five days a week (for six consecutive weeks) as well as implement one healthy eating habit each week. Since First Lady Michelle Obama kicked off the challenge, 1.7 million Americans have earned the awards certificate. I'd like you to take the PALA challenge this year! To learn more and sign up, go to www.presidentschallenge.org/donnarichardsonjoyner/.

It's all about attitude. If your attitude toward fitness and getting healthy is positive, you'll look forward to physical activity and find the time—no matter how busy you are—to fit in fitness. Pastor Joyce Meyer says, "The great thing about an attitude is that it's yours, and you can change it." So I'm asking you to change your attitude today and get excited about movement. Hip, hip, hooray!

9

Passport to Live

Ever had one of those mornings? Well, I was having one. I was supposed to get up and prepare for an upcoming speaking engagement, and I just couldn't get motivated. I was facing a challenge, feeling discouraged, and simply wanted to stay in bed and call in sick. But, as I lay there in my bed, my thoughts drifted from myself to Joyce.

When I met Joyce, she weighed about 500 pounds and was essentially bedridden. She was able to move only from her bed to a wheelchair and back to bed. She hadn't been able to walk in some time, and she desperately wanted to walk again and live a normal life. At only thirty-eight years of age, her obesity had forced her to live in a nursing home. I thought about the progress we had made over the past several months—she had lost 76 pounds, had given her life back to God, and was on track to walking again. I thought, "Joyce would give anything to be able to get out of bed and walk, and here I am lying in bed, feeling sorry for myself."

After a minute or two of that revelation sinking in, I climbed out of bed and declared, "I may be in pain, but I am going anyway! I may be stressed, but I'm going anyway. I may be tired, but I'm going

anyway!" You see, I realized that it wasn't about me. It didn't matter how I felt or what I wanted to do; it was so much bigger than that. When you realize that it's not about you, you go anyway. You make a way! That's what this journey is all about.

Many times the lessons we learn while helping others affect us for a lifetime. Because of experiences like the one I had with Joyce, I have become a better person and a better servant. Do you remember that famous scene from *How the Grinch Stole Christmas*, when the Grinch finally realizes that Christmas isn't about all the materialistic stuff but instead about loving, giving, and serving? The Grinch's eyes light up, he smiles, and then his heart grows three sizes larger? Well, I've never been much of a grinch, but even my big heart grows a little bigger every time I serve someone like Joyce,

---

SWEET TWEET

Celebrate every day U are in the land of the living, for in Christ it's about giving.

Love from your soul. Be BOLD!

> ## DONNAMITE SOUND BITE
>
> Donna is here as a guiding light; just remember to live right. You heard it from Coach Donnamite!

and I learn another lesson of the heart. Life can be challenging at times, but when you help people who cannot help themselves, it brings joy to your heart. When is the last time you did something for somebody else without expecting anything in return? Do you have a servant's heart? A true servant serves to the best of his or her ability, even when nobody is watching. It's not about your glory; it's about God's glory.

Sure, you want to lose weight and live a life of optimum health, but it's much bigger than that, isn't it? You want to be a better you so you can be a better spouse, a better parent, a better friend, a better employee—just a better human being! When you look at it from a holistic perspective, you realize the importance of being a good steward of your body, your temple. It's so much bigger! Self-improvement starts with you, but it continues with you helping and serving others.

Part of that self-improvement process involves opening yourself up to new experiences, new places, and new people. By doing so, you can broaden your mind and give yourself a new perspective. Bishop T. D. Jakes often says, "If you're the smartest person in your circle, it's time to get a new circle." I would have to agree. If you've been going to the same places with the same people and telling the same stories for most of your life, break out. Enlarge your vision. It's time to meet new people and learn new things. Sometimes we shut people out because they talk differently or move differently or think differently than we do, but when we shy away from those people, we miss out on so much. Step outside your comfort zone and embrace learning about other people. It will help you to grow. You might even learn a new language. That will definitely open up more opportunities to live an enriched and diverse life.

I believe in learning a new language so much that I challenged my godson to do just that when he was in college. I told him that if he did, I would pay for him to explore another country. He had the best chances: he dated a young Hispanic woman for a few years, and then he dated an Italian woman for four years after that, but he never took advantage of those personal, loving, 24/7 language tutors. He didn't learn another language, and he didn't get the prize. What is up with that? The good news is that he realized his missed opportunity. He travels to a different country every year and has now learned another language.

Birthday Wishes

My fiftieth birthday just passed, and I find myself pondering life and setting new goals. I've always been motivated and driven, but as I pass these milestones on my personal journey, it urges me to take inventory of my life. I think about where I've been, where I'm going, and what I have yet to accomplish.

Pastor A. R. Bernard of Brooklyn's Christian Cultural Center once said, "Growing older is automatic. Growing wiser is a choice." Can I get a big "amen"? One way to grow wiser is to expand one's horizons, and I've been traveling the world over the past twenty-five years. In fact, by my fiftieth birthday celebration, I had accomplished another of my goals: to visit all fifty states, fifty countries, and seven continents. (I have also crocheted over fifty afghans for loved ones, those who inspire me, and breast cancer survivors.) I love traveling. It educates you about people, cultures, and the world beyond your immediate surroundings. I've been privileged to do missionary work in Africa, Cuba, Haiti, South Africa, and Mexico, to name a few. I'll never forget traveling through a Third World country and watching the kids play on their rooftops. It was the safest place to play, since stray gunfire often plagued their city streets. I also remember the devastation that I saw during my missionary trip to Haiti. To this day, Haitians are living outdoors, with four poles and plastic coverings as their shelters. Many of them have no water, no electricity, and no food—just the clothes on their backs. But when I looked into their eyes, I saw strength, resilience, and hope.

That's what travel will do for you—it will give you an appreciation of your life. It gives you empathy, compassion, and an understanding of how to help those in need and contribute to making this world a better place. I know I've been blessed to be able to travel, and I want to share that blessing with others. The number 5 represents grace. For my fiftieth birthday gift, I took a group to Africa to educate, empower, and expose them to another country. Just as it did for me, this experience showed them the world through a different lens.

Growing and Giving

I've been keeping that "move to live, move to give" attitude alive in my spirit. I have a new vision for the next half century of my life: to visit fifty more countries, sowing seeds everywhere I go. You too can give back with the smallest of gestures, yet those small gestures bring big blessings. For example, when I travel I meet a lot of soldiers being deployed or returning from combat. I always carry thank-you cards for them. In those cards, I write some scripture and insert a little cash, just to tell them how much I appreciate all they have done and continue to do for our country. Several members of my family have served in the military, so I have a deep respect and gratitude for all servicemen and -women who sacrifice themselves for our country.

Think about ways to use your talent and resources to help others. One of my hobbies is crocheting and knitting. I crochet shawls and skullcaps, package them with scripture, and give

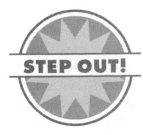

You are equipped with the essential tools you need to step out, be a better you, and accomplish something greater than you.

I challenge you:

- Love with every beat of your heart . . .

- Reach beyond what you can see or touch . . .

- Give more than you've given . . .

- Believe beyond what you can imagination . . .

- Live and flow in the rhythm of LIFE . . .

them to women going through radiation treatment and chemotherapy. You may say, "Well, Donna, that's great that you can do that, but I don't have any extra money to give to anyone." That's okay. There are other ways to give back.

I was once in the Chicago airport around Christmastime, and an ice storm hit the area. Needless to say, nobody was leaving that airport, and everyone was griping and moaning and complaining. People piled onto cots that lined the sides of every aisle while others rushed to whatever restaurant was open in hopes of finding a bit of food for the long night ahead. It was an atmosphere of anger, depression, and ugliness. On one side of me,

a man was cursing out an airline employee, and on the other side, a weary mother was letting her baby boy have it. It was crazy! Just then, the last flight to come in for the night deplaned, and off walked about thirty soldiers who had been serving in Iraq and were desperately trying to make it home for the holidays. As they walked into the airport, something magical happened. The complaining and moaning and ugliness subsided. All at once everyone stood up and began applauding these men and women in uniform. They were humbled by the intense and heartfelt show of gratitude. We were all moved. That didn't cost anyone anything, yet that small gesture of appreciation touched those soldiers' hearts and affected everyone there.

I once heard a pastor on TV challenge everyone to perform a selfless act of gratitude every single day. He suggested that whenever you see a firefighter or a police officer in a restaurant, tell your waitperson that you want to anonymously pick up that public servant's check. I thought it was a great idea! Another thing you can do that doesn't cost very much but sends a really big message of love is to pay for the car behind you at a drive-through window. Some people call this "paying it forward," but I like to call it "moving to give." Do the right thing and be a blessing! When God blows you sugar from heaven, share that sugar with others. Blow kisses of love, life, happiness, and hope to everyone you encounter.

Our family tries to blow those kisses of love every Christmas Eve: we select a local women's shelter and play Santa's helpers for the night. We shower them with food, gifts, good cheer, and lots of love. We've been doing this for the past ten years, and I look forward to it every holiday season. We do a similar outreach of love at a women's shelter every Valentine's Day. Why? Because helping others is an honor, and because I believe that to whom much is given, much will be required.

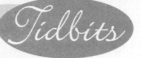

TRANSFORMATION Tidbits

- "Growing older is automatic. Growing wiser is a choice."—Pastor A. R. Bernard

- Many times the lessons we learn while helping others affect us for a lifetime.

- Traveling educates you about people, cultures, and the world beyond your immediate surroundings.

- When God blows you sugar from heaven, share that sugar with others. Blow kisses of love, life, happiness, and hope to everyone you encounter.

- You may be facing adversity, but you have to push forward to give birth to new beginnings.

- The difficulty you're facing right now may be the very thing that thrusts you on to your ultimate destiny.

- Faith and gratitude are the power twins of life.

Pastor Paula White once said, "The end goal of locating yourself is to give away the authentic you—to use your talents and abilities to benefit others and to bless a needy world." That's exactly what my friend Cheryl "Action" Jackson did. She saw a need, knew she would be the perfect person to fill that need, and set out to do just that. You see, Cheryl grew up knowing what it was like to go hungry, and later she experienced the torment of wondering how she would feed her family. She understood the phrase "surviving, not thriving" all too well. Even though she was living in Plano, a very affluent city near Dallas, Texas, she still struggled. And she knew she wasn't alone. So, in April 2007 Cheryl decided to bless a needy world. Taking items from her kitchen, she opened Minnie's Food Pantry, named after her mother, Minnie Ewing. That first day, she fed three families, and within the first month, she had fifty-two families turning to her for meals. To date, Minnie's Food Pantry has fed more than 93,000 people and distributed more than 1.3 million pounds of food, but it all began with one woman who saw a need, believed she could make a difference, and stepped out on faith. Every day she is somebody's miracle. When is the last time you were somebody's miracle?

From Test to Testimony

God will use whatever you've come through to make a difference in somebody else's life. Listen, I've been through hell and high water, and that's why I can confidently say to you, if you put your faith in God, he will bring you through. When you have faith in your Creator and faith in yourself, your thinking should be "I will overcome and be victorious." You should be able to look back at how far you've come and shout, "The best is yet to come!" Your theme song should be like the words of the Pointer Sisters' hit: "I know darn well we can work it out. Oh yes, we can, I know we can can. Yes, we can can." Yes, you can can! I know you can can!

I couldn't help people like Joyce if I hadn't waged my own battles and won. I couldn't write this book and encourage you to strive for total health in your mind, spirit, and body if I hadn't been knocked down and gotten back up. I'm not just talking about a faith that somebody else has put to the test; I'm telling you that I've put my faith to the test and I've come out victorious! In other words, you may be down, but you're not out. You may be facing adversity, but you have to push forward to give birth to new beginnings. And the difficulty you may be facing right now may be the very thing that thrusts you on to your ultimate destiny. There is a purpose for our pain . . . just ask Pastor Darlene Bishop.

You may have heard Pastor Darlene share her testimony on her TBN program, *Sisters*. The Creator called Pastor Darlene to preach when she was only fourteen years old, but she didn't become an international minister and bestselling author until she battled breast cancer at age forty-one and received a supernatural healing from God. She tells of the morning her tumor-ridden breast was bleeding into the bathroom sink; the pain was so great it actually took her breath away. Still, she looked into that bathroom mirror and with everything in her said, "God, what's going on in this body doesn't change the fact that you are still the Healer. I will believe it and preach it until the very last breath leaves my body." She received her miracle that very morning. After she stood in the face of a terminal diagnosis and proclaimed God as her Healer, she had a powerful testimony.

And that testimony has touched the hearts of thousands. Today when naysayers write, "God doesn't heal anymore," she can stand up and proclaim, "Yes, he does! I have a testimony!" You can't tell Pastor Darlene Bishop that the Creator isn't real. You can't tell her that the Creator doesn't heal. She has experienced his healing, his love, and his deliverance in her life. Her test has become her greatest testimony. Will yours?

Faith and Gratitude— the Power Twins

Inspirational speaker Iyanla Vanzant once said, "I had to listen within to conquer without. Faith kept my heart open and allowed me gratitude." I love that quote so much, because I believe that faith and gratitude are the power twins of life. Because of your faith, you can be grateful for all the good things in your life today and all the blessings to come. You won't doubt there are blessings on the way; instead, you'll be on the lookout for them. No matter what the state of your well-being today, you'll look through the windows of faith and see that future version of yourself better than before.

You may not be able to walk in a 5K right now. You may be totally overwhelmed and completely stressed out at this moment. But you have to envision yourself the way you want to be. It doesn't matter what you're facing today, if you have faith that you're going to make it through. You can have gratitude in your heart for all the good things in your life now and all the fantastic things in your future. That faith–gratitude connection is strong, and it's important that you possess both as you continue along this road.

Pause for a minute and ponder these questions: What is your greatest adversity? What is your gift that needs to be developed? What dreams do you need to birth? What is stopping you from cherishing every day and living life to the fullest?

Maybe you're like Joyce, who is working her way back to walking again and regaining her independence. Or maybe you're like Pastor Darlene, who had to face her foe head-on and believe she would come through victorious. Or maybe you're like me: you've come to a milestone in your life and you're ready to do more, give more, and be more. Or maybe for the first time in your life you realize that your existence on this earth is for a greater purpose, and you're ready to achieve all of those things on your vision tree. I don't know your exact situation but I do know this: you are ready to move out, move up, and move on. It wasn't by accident that you picked up this book; it was divine intervention. And now you have the mental, spiritual, and physical tools to transform your health and your life.

Oprah Winfrey once said, "There is a vision for my life that is greater than my imagination can hold." Your vision for your life should be that great too. Life is constantly shifting, but if you continue having the courage to face it, the perseverance and patience to get things done, and the faith to believe in the impossible, you'll be unstoppable. You are moving beyond what you think you can achieve and stepping into your destiny today. This isn't just about you. This isn't just about me. We are all in this together! Be a witness to fitness, and experience the journey to newness and wholeness in your health.

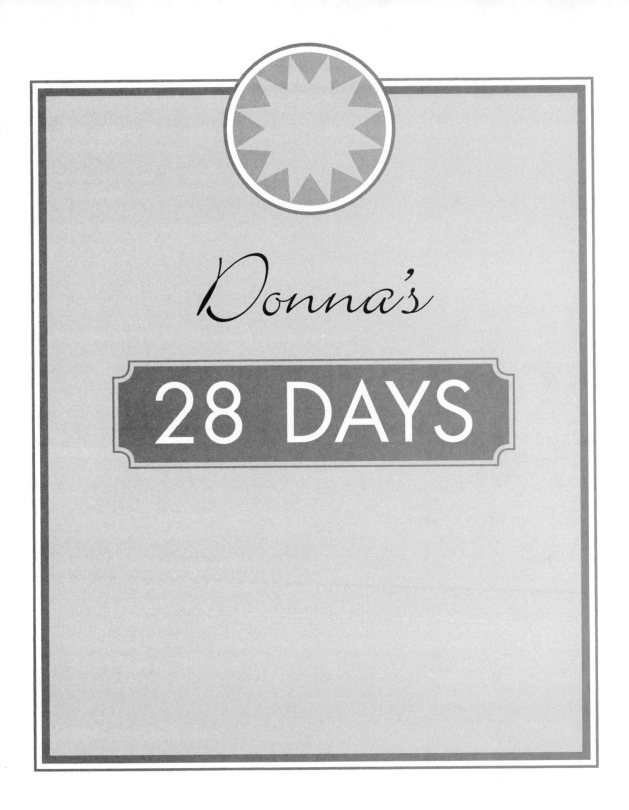

3-Day Jump Start

The 3-day Jump Start program will provide you with shakes, vegetables, and salads.

FRUIT LIST   *Approximately 80 calories*

Apple, 1 medium	Grapes, 1 cup	Papaya, ½ small	Strawberries, sliced,
Banana, ½	Kiwi, 1 medium	Peach, 1 medium	1 cup
Blackberries, ¾ cup	Mango, ½ small	Pear, 1 medium	Tangerines, 2 small
Blueberries, ¾ cup	Melon, 1 cup	Pineapple, 1 cup	
Boysenberries, 1 cup	Nectarine, 1 medium	Plums, 2 small	
Grapefruit, ½ large	Orange, 1 medium	Raspberries, 1 cup	

SALAD LIST

Endive, Lettuce (any kind except iceberg), Spinach

VEGETABLE LIST

Arugula	Brussels sprouts	Collard greens	Mushrooms
Asparagus	Cabbage	Cucumber	Parsley
Bell pepper	Cauliflower	Green onions, chopped	Radishes
Bok choy	Celery	Green string beans	Snap peas
Broccoli	Chard	Kale	Snow peas

NUTS AND SEEDS LIST   *Approximately 100 calories (all raw)*

Almonds, 17 whole nuts	Flaxseed, ground, 3 tablespoons	Peanuts, 17 whole nuts	Sunflower seeds (hulled), 2 tablespoons
Chia seeds, 2 tablespoons	Hempseed, shelled, 2 tablespoons	Pecans, 10 halves	Walnuts, 8 halves
		Sesame seeds, 2 tablespoons	

JUMP-START VINAIGRETTE

4 tablespoons extra-virgin olive oil
2 tablespoons balsamic vinegar
2 teaspoons Dijon mustard (or to taste)
Pepper to taste

Directions: Add all ingredients to a sealable container and shake it up, baby!

Nutrition facts for 2 tablespoons: 170 calories, 0 grams protein, 2 grams carbohydrates, 188 grams fat, 0 grams fiber

Be Faithful

I have come that they may have life, and that
they may have it more abundantly.
—JOHN 10:10

Be Grateful

JOY'S STORY

Turning 40 was a monumental event for my friend Joy. On that day, she decided to embrace the calling of copastoring the Potter's House of Denver. She also decided to take the first steps toward a strong, healthy spirit, soul, and body. Joy started her journey doing a 21-day Daniel Fast. She said, "You can get on the treadmill every day, but if you don't believe in your heart and mind, the transformation on the outside won't happen. Change has to happen from within."

Another turning point happened for Joy when I met with her in Miami. I invited her to go shopping with me. She admitted later that she was embarrassed to shop with me because I was a size 2, and she wasn't. That same fear kept her out of the gym. She didn't want to work out with fit, sculpted bodies all around her. Finally, one day, she said, "Enough! I am facing my fears!"

Today, Joy has lost more than 40 pounds. She quit making excuses and started making progress. She faced her fears and allowed the Lord to help her in this weight-loss journey, and now she is leading the way for many others.

Be Positive

Stop making excuses and start making progress. It's time to face your fears and step out in faith. This is your time to shine!

Be Fruitful

Day 1

BREAKFAST: Shake

In a blender, combine 1 serving of Greenberry, Chocolate, or Tropical Strawberry Shakeology (or 6 ounces of any low-sugar protein powder) with 8 to 10 ounces of water and 1 serving from both the fruit list and the nuts and seeds list. Add as much ice as you want. Whirl until blended.

BONUS SNACK: Spread Out the Wealth!

If you want to leave the fruit or nuts and seeds out of either your breakfast or lunch smoothie, you can enjoy them here as a snack.

LUNCH: Shake

In a blender, combine 1 serving of Greenberry, Chocolate, or Tropical Strawberry Shakeology (or 6 ounces of any low-sugar protein powder) with 8 to 10 ounces of water and 1 serving from the fruit list only. Add as much ice as you want. Whirl until blended.

DINNER: Salad

In a large bowl, combine 1 ingredient from the salad list and 3 ingredients from the vegetable list. Don't worry about amounts. We've populated the lists with super-healthy, super-low-calorie options, so you could eat yourself silly and probably still stay below 200 calories. Add 2 tablespoons Jump-Start Vinaigrette or a similar olive oil–based dressing, and you're good to go.

SNACK: Shake

In a blender, combine 1 serving of Greenberry, Chocolate, or Tropical Strawberry Shakeology (or 6 ounces of any low-sugar protein powder) with 8 to 10 ounces of water. Add as much ice as you want. Whirl until blended.

Be Joyful

SONG OF THE DAY: "Faith" by George Michael

Be Fit

WARM-UP: 3–5 minutes
CARDIO: 30–60 minutes
STRENGTH TRAINING: Indoor Boot Camp
STRETCH: 3–5 minutes

Indoor Boot Camp Workout

High Knee Lifts

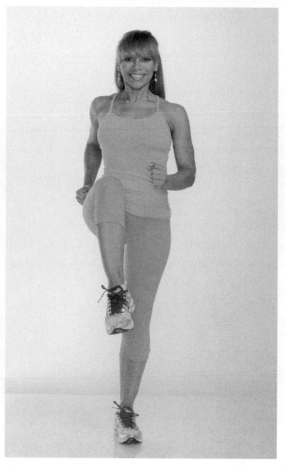

Exercise 1
Stand tall with your abs tightened and your arms bent at your waist. Start with alternating high knee lifts. Perform for 1 minute.

Alternating Front Leg Raises

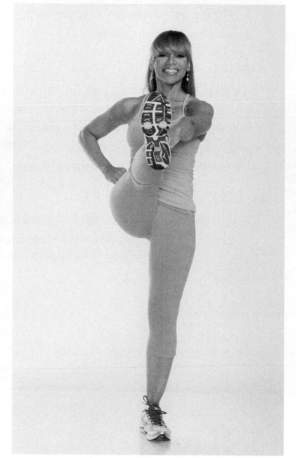

Exercise 2
Stand tall with your abs contracted, your arms bent, and your hands on your hips. Alternate leg lifts to the front while reaching toward your leg with the opposite arm. Perform for 1 minute.

Trunk Twist

Exercise 3

Stand tall with your feet hip-width apart, your arms bent with elbows to the sides and your fingertips touching the back of your head. Contract your abs and lift your knee up, rotating your torso to the side with your shoulder pointed toward your knee. Return to the starting position and repeat on the other side. Perform for 1 minute.

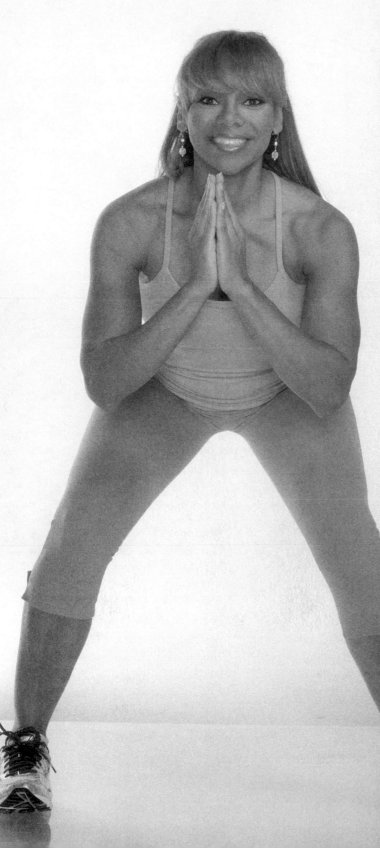

Squat Jumps

Exercise 4

Start in a squat position with your feet more than hip-width apart, your arms bent, and elbows at your sides. Jump, bringing your feet together while you remain in a squat position. Jump, with your feet coming together and then apart, for 1 minute.

Alternating Side Kick

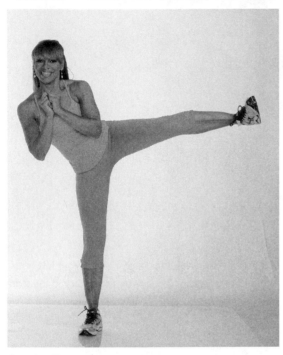

Exercise 5

Stand tall, with your abs contracted, your feet slightly apart, and your arms bent in front of your chest. Lean to one side and extend the opposite leg out to the side in a side kick motion. Return to the starting position. Alternate from side to side. Perform for 1 minute.

Side Rotational Plank

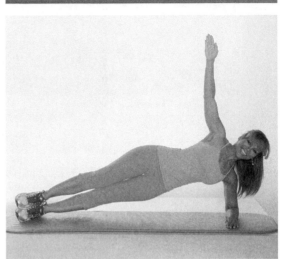

Exercise 6

Lying facedown, lift up into a plank position on elbows and toes with your body in a straight line. Rotate your torso, lifting up on your left arm, and raise your right arm straight overhead. Hold for 3 seconds and return to plank position parallel to the floor. Perform, alternating sides, for 1 minute.

Back Extensions

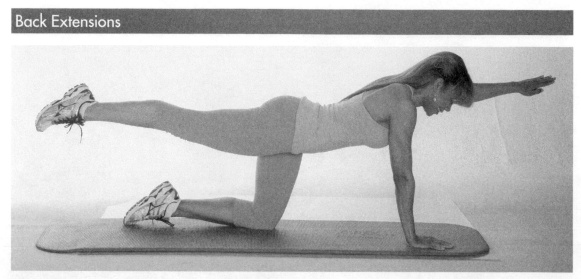

Exercise 7

Start on hands and knees, hands under shoulders and knees under hips. Simultaneously extend your left arm forward and your right leg back so that they are parallel to the floor. Hold for 3 seconds and return to the start position. Do 16 reps, then switch to the other side and repeat. Perform, alternating sides, for 1 minute.

Roll-Up

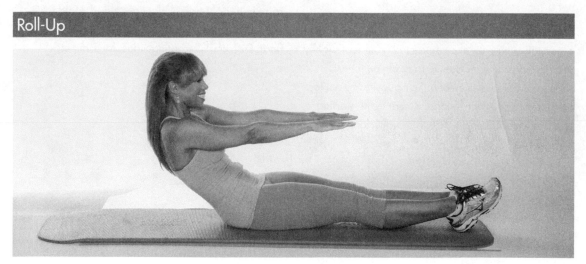

Exercise 8

Lie on your back with your legs straight and your arms extended above your head. Contract your abs and roll up to a seated position with your arms straight in front of you at chest level and your feet resting on the floor. Then slowly roll back down to the starting position with your feet remaining on the floor. Perform for 1 minute.

REPEAT CIRCUIT 1–3 TIMES.

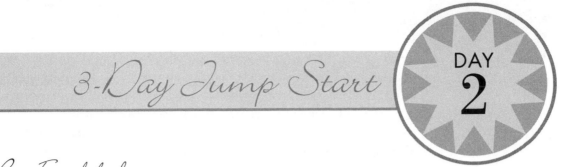

Be Faithful

For as the body without the spirit is dead,
so faith without works is dead also.
—JAMES 2:26

Be Grateful

LENELL'S STORY

Lenell W. went from 360 lbs. to 180 lbs. in six years.

I was a Hurricane Katrina victim, and I had to relocate and start all over in an unfamiliar place. However, that was not my biggest challenge. My biggest challenge was that I was obese and depressed. But I had not given up hope. Donna was the first person to embrace me and let me know that there was more in me than what the eye could see.

I told God that I didn't want to die an obese woman. I didn't want it on my death certificate that I died due to complications of obesity. What people don't understand about the really obese is that you're like a prisoner in your own body. It's like a trap. I didn't feel as if the person in the mirror matched who I was on the inside because there was so much more to me—and there had to be more to life. I was crying out for help, and God answered my prayers by sending me a health angel, Donna.

I used to be a person who couldn't walk a few steps without gasping for breath. Now my energy level is high. I work at the airport as a personal care assistant, helping people who are in wheelchairs. I walk miles and miles every day. I never could have done this job at my former weight.

It is ironic that I am now a manager at a restaurant, so I am surrounded by food. Food has been my biggest challenge for most of my life. Yet I am disciplined and stick to my nutritional plan. I eat a lot of grilled fish, grilled shrimp, and grilled chicken. My favorite vegetables are green beans, spinach, and salads.

I'm thankful for angels sent by God. The first was Oprah Winfrey, who started me on my weight-loss program, where I lost 100 pounds. Oprah planted the seed, but ultimately I had to make up my mind to live and not die. My second angel is Donna R. Joyner. I had been praying that somehow God would allow me to meet her. Not only did I meet her, but she helped me lose 79 more pounds. In working with her I also strengthened my walk with God, and I came to believe I could do all things through Christ. I don't care what anyone says—I'm her one soldier and I'm going out on the road to share the gospel of being a witness to fitness.

I will forever be indebted to my angels. I have lost 180 pounds and have taken control of my health. I'm dedicated to helping and inspiring others. I am on a crusade to stop obesity, and I am here to tell you that if I can do it, you can, too.

Sincerely,

Lenell

Be Positive

Have the courage to exceed your expectations and have the faith to be fearless when faced with the unknown.

Be Fruitful

Day 2

BREAKFAST: Shake

In a blender, combine 1 serving of Greenberry, Chocolate, or Tropical Strawberry Shakeology (or 6 ounces of any low-sugar protein powder) with 8 to 10 ounces of water and 1 serving from both the fruit list and the nuts and seeds list. Add as much ice as you want. Whirl until blended.

BONUS SNACK: Spread Out the Wealth!

If you want to leave the fruit or nuts and seeds out of either your breakfast or lunch smoothie, you can enjoy them here as a snack.

LUNCH: Shake

In a blender, combine 1 serving of Greenberry, Chocolate, or Tropical Strawberry Shakeology (or 6 ounces of any low-sugar protein powder) with 8 to 10 ounces of water and 1 serving from the fruit list only. Add as much ice as you want. Whirl until blended.

DINNER: Salad

In a large bowl, combine 1 ingredient from the salad list and 3 ingredients from the vegetable list. Don't worry about amounts. We've populated the lists with super-healthy, super-low-calorie options, so you could eat yourself silly and probably still stay below 200 calories.

Add 2 tablespoons Jump-Start Vinaigrette or a similar olive oil–based dressing, and you're good to go.

SNACK: Shake

In a blender, combine 1 serving of Greenberry, Chocolate, or Tropical Strawberry Shakeology (or 6 ounces of any low-sugar protein powder) with 8 to 10 ounces of water. Add as much ice as you want. Whirl until blended.

Be Joyful

SONG OF THE DAY: "The Power of Love" by Huey Lewis and the News

Be Fit

WARM-UP: 3–5 minutes
CARDIO: 30–60 minutes
STRENGTH TRAINING: Bootylicious
STRETCH: 3–5 minutes

Bootylicious Workout

Bent-Leg Hip Extension

Start on your hands and knees, your hands under your shoulders, your knees under your hips, your abs contracted, and your back flat. Bring one knee toward your chest (Position A), contract your buttocks, and extend your leg back (Position B). Return to the starting position. Perform 16 reps, then switch to the other leg and repeat.

Position A

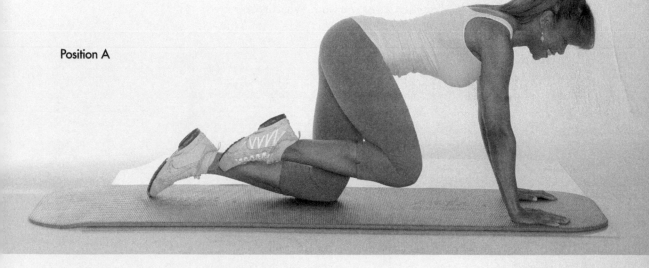

Position B

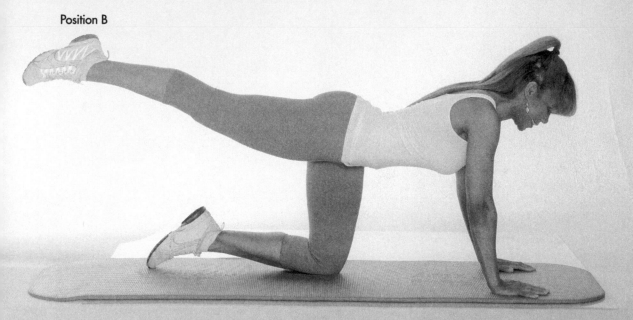

Straight-Leg Hip Extension

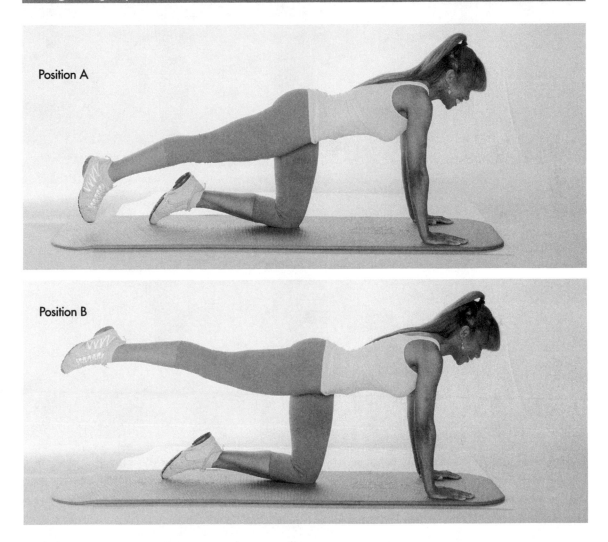

Position A

Position B

Start on your hands and knees, your hands under your shoulders, your knees under your hips, your abs contracted, and your back flat. Extend your leg straight behind you, touching your toe to the ground (Position A), contract your buttocks, and lift your leg up (Position B). Lower your leg to the start position. Perform 16 reps, then switch to the other leg and repeat.

Hip Extension Crossover

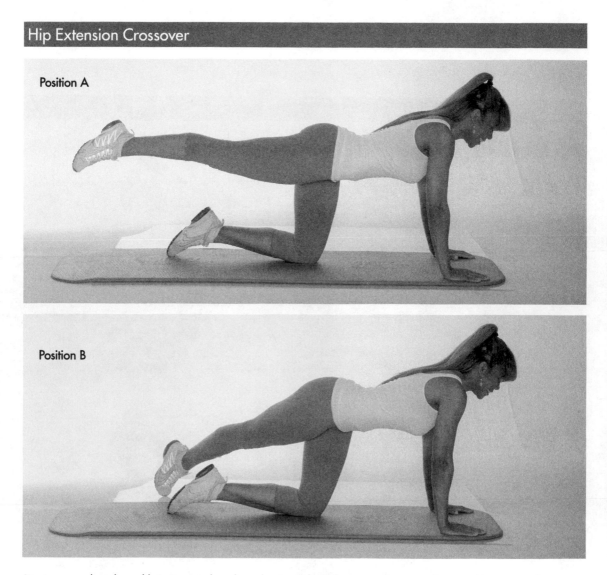

Position A

Position B

Start on your hands and knees, your hands under your shoulders, your knees under your hips, your abs contracted, and your back flat. Start by extending one leg back (Position A). Keeping your hips still, cross the leg over your bent knee, touching your toe to the ground (Position B). Return to the starting position. Perform 16 reps, then switch to the other leg and repeat.

Quadruped

Get down on your hands and knees, your hands under your shoulders, your knees under your hips, your abs contracted, and your back flat. Lift your bent right knee out to the side (Position A), then lower it back down. Lift the same bent leg back and up behind you (Position B), then lower it back down. Perform 16 reps. On the last bent-leg lift, hold the raised position and pulse up (contract) for 32 counts, then lower your leg to the start position. Switch legs and repeat.

REPEAT CIRCUIT 1–3 TIMES.

Position A

Position B

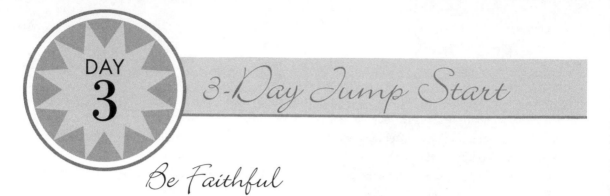

Be Faithful

*What? Know ye not that your body is the temple
of the Holy Ghost which is in you, which ye have
of God, and ye are not your own?*
—1 CORINTHIANS 6:19

Be Grateful

ANTHONY'S STORY

*By now you know that I think the right mind-set is the key to success. You also
have to be relentless and have the tenacity to go after what you want. Once in a
while a story comes along that is the perfect example of this. I recently read about
a young wrestler named Anthony Robles who was born with just one leg. But
Robles hasn't allowed his disability to hold him back.*

*Robles had an amazing undefeated record (36–0) in the 125-pound class his
senior year at Arizona State University, winning the NCAA title in Philadelphia
in 2011. Robles got a standing ovation after the win and then stood on the podium
with his crutches. "My mom told me that God made me for a reason, and that
reason was wrestling," Robles told USA Today.*

*Anthony claims to draw inspiration from letters sent by kids and adults
saying they're motivated by what he has done. I was incredibly moved by this
young man. He believes that he is a champion, the best at what he does, and he
puts no limits on his potential. In Anthony's mind, he is not disabled. Although
he has a physical limitation, it does not hinder him from being all he can be.
Anthony's outlook on life supersedes any obstacles or challenges he could ever face.
He has never stopped striving, never stopped fighting—and he is achieving the
ultimate success!*

Be Positive

Your body—you can't replace it or trade it in.
Treasure your body with respect, love, and care.

Be Fruitful

Day 3

BREAKFAST: Shake

In a blender, combine 1 serving of Greenberry, Chocolate, or Tropical Strawberry Shakeology (or 6 ounces of any low-sugar protein powder) with 8 to 10 ounces of water and 1 serving from both the fruit list and the nuts and seeds list. Add as much ice as you want. Whirl until blended.

BONUS SNACK: Spread Out the Wealth!

If you want to leave the fruit or nuts and seeds out of either your breakfast or lunch smoothie, you can enjoy them here as a snack.

LUNCH: Shake

In a blender, combine 1 serving of Greenberry, Chocolate, or Tropical Strawberry Shakeology (or 6 ounces of any low-sugar protein powder) with 8 to 10 ounces of water and 1 serving from the fruit list only. Add as much ice as you want. Whirl until blended.

DINNER: Salad

In a large bowl, combine 1 ingredient from the salad list and 3 ingredients from the vegetable list. Don't worry about amounts. We've populated the lists with super-healthy, super-low-calorie options, so you could eat yourself silly and probably still stay below 200 calories.

Add 2 tablespoons Jump-Start Vinaigrette or a similar olive oil–based dressing and you're good to go.

SNACK: Shake

In a blender, combine 1 serving of Greenberry, Chocolate, or Tropical Strawberry Shakeology (or 6 ounces of any low-sugar protein powder) with 8 to 10 ounces of water. Add as much ice as you want. Whirl until blended.

Be Joyful

SONG OF THE DAY: "Flood" by Jars of Clay

Be Fit

WARM-UP: 3–5 minutes
CARDIO: 30–60 minutes
STRENGTH TRAINING: Best Bosom
STRETCH: 3–5 minutes

Best Bosom Workout

Modified Push-Up

Start on your hands and knees with your feet up, your abs tight, and your back straight (Position A). Bend your elbows and lower your chest to the floor (Position B). Push through the palms of your hands and straighten your arms to the starting position. Perform 15 reps.

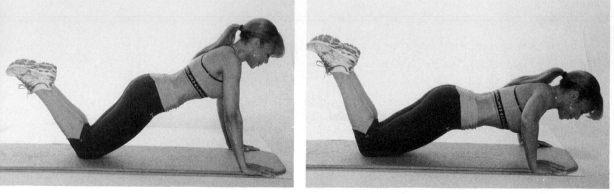

Position A   Position B

Chest Press

Lie on your back with your knees bent, your feet flat on the ground, your elbows bent, and weights in your hands (Position A). Contract your chest muscles and press the weights toward the ceiling by straightening your arms (Position B). Return to the starting position. Perform 15 reps.

Optional: Put a couple of pillows under your head and back.

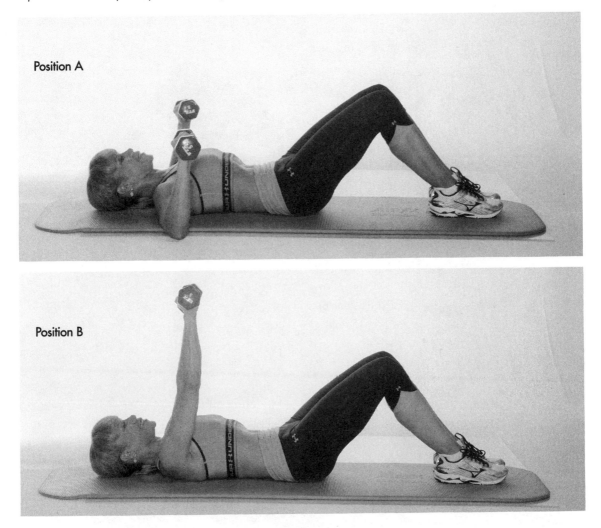

Position A

Position B

Chest Fly

Start in the same position as the last exercise. Hold weights in your hands and extend your arms to the sides, keeping them rounded (Position A). Contract your chest muscles and bring the weights together above your chest (Position B). Return to the starting position. Perform 15 reps.

Optional: Put pillows or folded towels under your head and back.

Position A

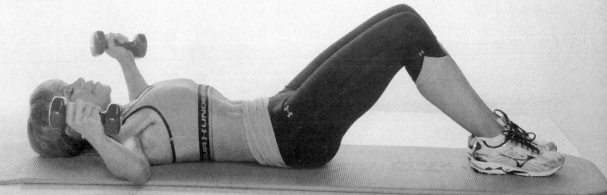

Position B

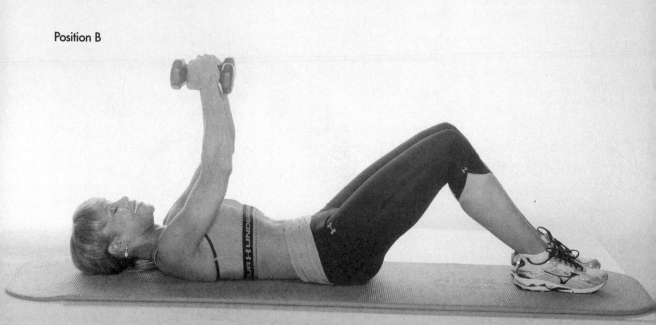

Walk Out and In Plank

Lie facedown on your stomach, then lift your body into a plank position, balancing on elbows and toes with your body in a straight line (Position A). Contract your abs, your chest, and your shoulder muscles. Walk your feet out to the sides and then back in for 30–60 seconds. Lower yourself back to the starting position. Perform 4–6 times.

REPEAT CIRCUIT 1–3 TIMES.

Position A

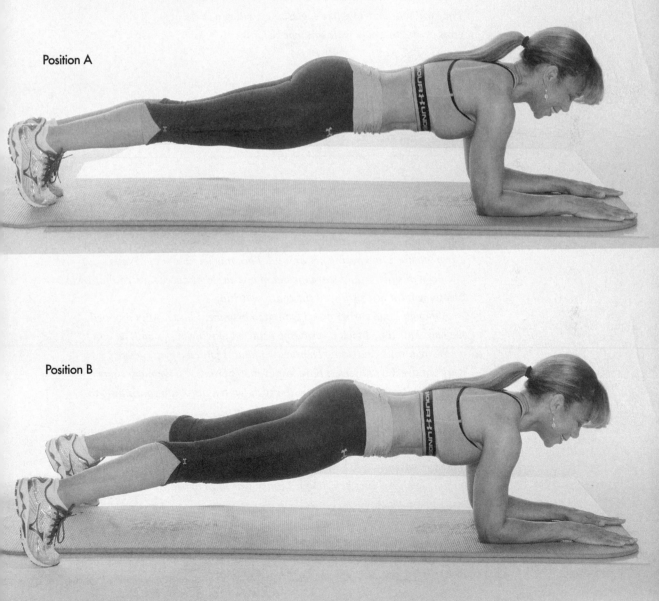

Position B

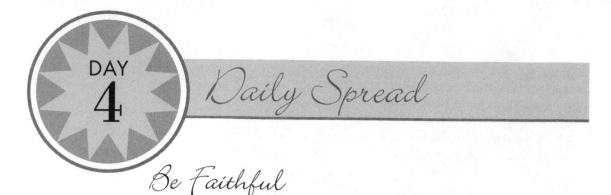

Be Faithful

But those who hope in the Lord will renew their strength.
They will soar on wings like eagles; they will run and not
grow weary, they will walk and not be faint.
—ISAIAH 40:31

Be Grateful

PETE'S STORY

Pete went from 300 lbs. to 270 lbs. in three months.

In 2011 my weight had escalated to about 300 pounds in a little less than a year's
time. When I'd play with my little girl, picking her up, carrying her up and
down the stairs, or chasing her around, I became terribly tired. Walking up just
one flight of stairs would leave me out of breath. My fiancée noticed that I was
breathing hard just sitting on the couch watching TV.

Although I had earlier asked Donna to help me, I had always dropped
the ball. This time I took it seriously. I started playing basketball, walking
on the treadmill, and doing Donna's workout. I joined a gym, where I now
work out five days a week. I have lost over 30 pounds, I have more energy, I
don't get as tired when playing with my daughter, and I am continuing to
lose weight.

Aside from becoming more physically active, I have learned about eating
healthier foods and controlling portion size. I started eating smaller portions and
no longer eat past 8:00 P.M. I increased my water intake and stopped snacking
on junk food. Another key change I made was to go to bed early, which helped me
avoid midnight cravings.

What I have learned in this process is that change takes patience and
time. This is a new lifestyle for me, and I now realize that I have to take steps
every day to become a healthier and happier person. Donna continues to

encourage me by telling me that I can do it, and she is giving me the inspiration to keep on truckin'.
Sincerely,
Pete

Be Positive

Take action today and go after all that your heart desires.
Be faithful, be fruitful, and be a fighter.

Be Fruitful

BREAKFAST: Green and White Omelet with Watermelon

In a nonstick skillet coated with cooking spray, make an omelet with 1 whole egg and 3 egg whites, filled with ½ cup steamed broccoli florets and 1 ounce soft goat cheese. Serve with 1 slice light-style wheat bread and 1 cup cubed watermelon.

305 calories, 26 grams protein, 27 grams carbohydrate,
11 grams fat, 5 grams fiber

SNACK: Lemon Berry Smoothie

In a blender, combine 1 scoop Greenberry Shakeology (or 6 ounces of any low-sugar protein powder), ⅓ cup lemon juice (*not* lemonade), 1 cup water, and 1 cup crushed ice.

150 calories, 17 grams protein, 17 grams carbohydrate,
1 gram fat, 3 grams fiber

LUNCH: Chicken and Hummus Wrap

On a 6-inch whole-wheat tortilla (about 100 calories), spread 3 tablespoons hummus, then layer 3 ounces grilled chicken breast cut in strips, 2 slices red onion, ¼ cup alfalfa sprouts, 2 slices ripe tomato, and ¼ cup shredded romaine lettuce. Roll, cut in half, and serve.

397 calories, 36 grams protein, 40 grams carbohydrate,
14 grams fat, 9 grams fiber

SNACK: Turkey and Carrots

1 ounce sliced white-meat turkey and 10 baby carrots, with ¼ cup hummus for dipping.

158 calories, 11 grams protein, 16 grams carbohydrate,
6 grams fat, 5 grams fiber

DINNER: Herb-Grilled Orange Roughy

On a preheated grill pan sprayed with cooking spray, grill a 5-ounce fillet of orange roughy (or white flaky fish of choice) brushed with 2 teaspoons olive oil. Season with salt, pepper, and ¼ cup fresh herbs. Serve with 1 cup green beans sautéed in 1 teaspoon olive oil and minced garlic, with ½ cup cooked brown rice.

For dessert: ½ cup cubed honeydew

415 calories, 30 grams protein, 49 grams carbohydrate,
15 grams fat, 6 grams fiber

Be Joyful

SONG OF THE DAY: "Crazy in Love" by Beyoncé

Be Fit

WARM-UP: 3–5 minutes
CARDIO: 30–60 minutes
STRENGTH TRAINING: Fab, Fierce, and Fun
STRETCH: 3–5 minutes

Fab, Fierce, and Fun Workout

Tricep Extension and Side Leg Lift

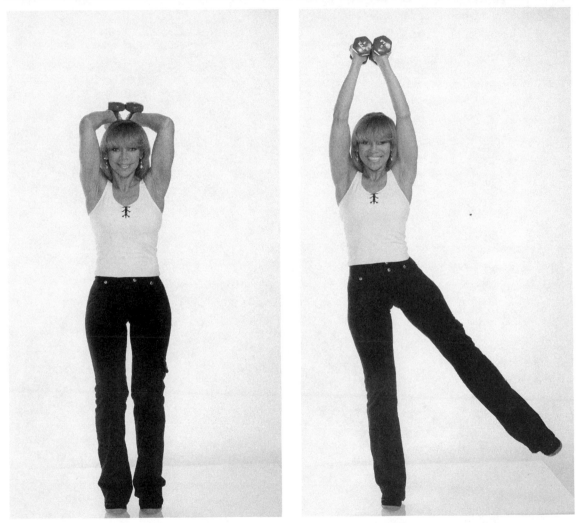

Position A

Position B

Stand with your feet hip-width apart, your arms bent back and held close to your ears, and weights in your hands. Lower your body to a demi-squat. This is your starting position (Position A). As you straighten your legs to a standing position, lift one leg to the side and raise your arms above your head. Lower yourself to the starting position and repeat the entire exercise. Perform 15 reps, then switch sides and repeat.

Lunge with Knee Lift and Twist

Stand with your feet slightly apart, holding weights at chest level. Step your right leg back into a lunge (Position A). Step up onto your left leg, lifting your right knee, contract your abdominals, and turn your upper body to the right (Position B). Perform 15 reps, then switch sides and repeat.

Position A

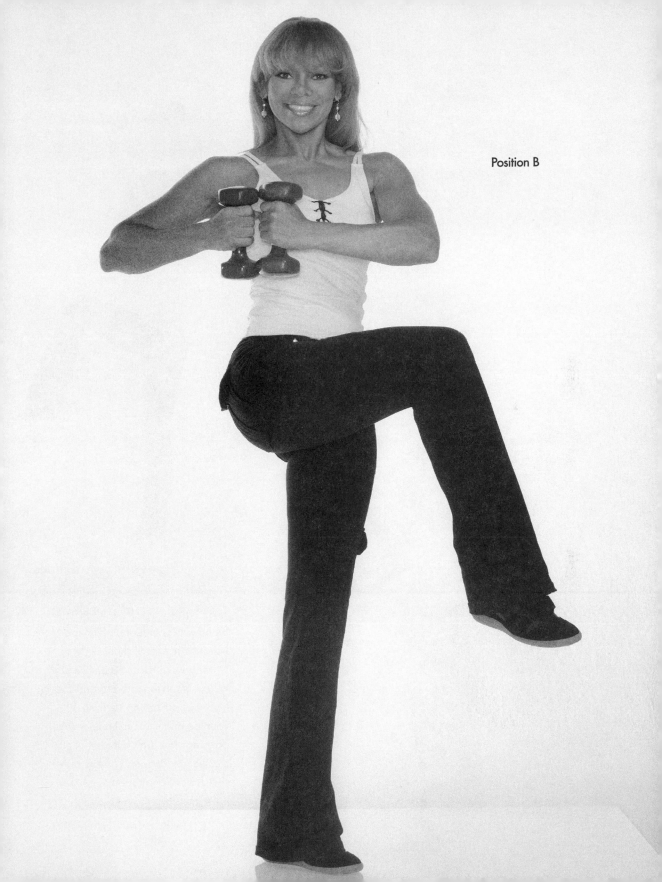

Position B

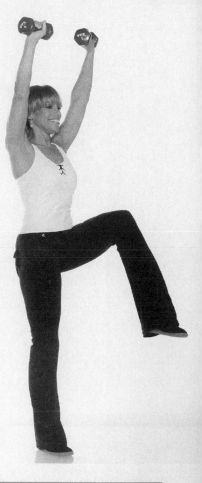

Position B

Position A

Side Lunge and Bicep Curl

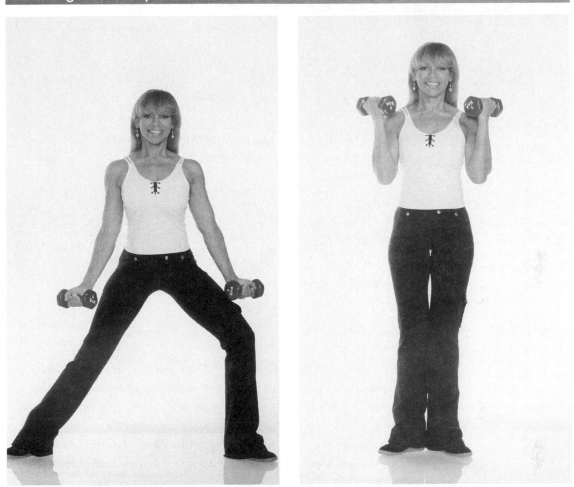

Position A   **Position B**

Stand with your feet slightly apart, arms alongside your body and weights in your hands. Step sideways into a lunge (Position A). As you return to the starting position, contract your biceps and lift the weights to shoulder level (Position B). Perform 15 reps, then repeat with the lunge on the other side.

REPEAT CIRCUIT 1–3 TIMES.

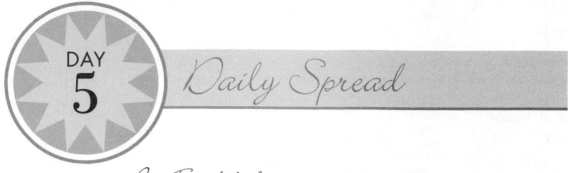

Be Faithful

And the LORD answered me, and said, Write the vision, and make it plain on tables, that he may run that reads it.

—HABAKKUK 2:2

Be Grateful

STEPHANIE'S STORY

Stephanie went from 218 lbs. to 178 lbs. in eight months.

The time is now to break hereditary strongholds, and it starts with me. I have two daughters and I didn't want them to see their mom as someone who had her life together spiritually but was letting her body break down. In addition, I mentor some girls in the church, and my goal was to show them that you can make changes and have wholeness in your life. I knew I couldn't be a good mentor if my health was a wreck. I made a choice to become healthier and to lead by example so that I would be a better role model for my daughters and mentees. In short, I made a decision to take better care of myself so I could take better care of others.

My family has a history of high blood pressure and diabetes. When I was pregnant with my last child, I had gestational diabetes during the last two months. I knew that if my health improved, I wouldn't have to rely anymore on the medication I was taking. I began following Donna's DVDs and also started eating smaller portions and stopped eating red meat. I now drink more water and avoid sodas. Usually my biggest meal is at lunch, and I don't have dinner any later than about 7:30 P.M.

I do my devotional every morning around five. I say my prayer, read scripture, and then sit there and let the words minister to me. I wait to hear God's voice through his word to empower and encourage me for the day. Then

I exercise, which keeps the worship experience going. I've lost 40 pounds, and I continue to nourish my body and soul. God is good!

Yours truly,

Stephanie

Be Positive

Use your willpower to fulfill your purpose and destiny in life. Don't give up, don't give in. Persevere!

Be Fruitful

BREAKFAST: Steel-Cut Oatmeal with Turkey Sausage

Cook 1 cup steel-cut oats in water. Top with ¼ cup skim milk and a pinch of ground cinnamon. Serve with 2 turkey sausage links.

297 calories, 21 grams protein, 29 grams carbohydrate, 11 grams fat, 4 grams fiber

SNACK: Figs and Cheese

2 small figs, sliced, with 2 tablespoons crumbled blue cheese and 1 ounce deli ham.

160 calories, 10 grams protein, 15 grams carbohydrate, 7 grams fat, 2.5 grams fiber

LUNCH: Cheddar Burger with Mixed Greens

Broil a 3-ounce ground sirloin burger on both sides until it's cooked through, then top with 1 ounce reduced-fat cheddar cheese and 2 slices red onion. Serve between 2 slices light-style wheat bread, with a small salad of mixed greens dressed with 2 tablespoons low-calorie Italian dressing (approximately 40 calories). Serve with ½ cup cubed cantaloupe.

398 calories, 35 grams protein, 41 grams carbohydrate, 12 grams fat, 7 grams fiber

SNACK: Cottage Cheese

⅓ cup low-fat (1% or 2%) cottage cheese topped with 1 tablespoon flaxseed and 1 tablespoon raisins.

140 calories, 10 grams protein, 14 grams carbohydrate, 5 grams fat, 3 grams fiber

DINNER: Lemon Chicken

Marinate a 3-ounce boneless, skinless chicken breast in lemon juice and olive oil. Bake at 375°F until cooked through (about 20 to 25 minutes). Serve with a small baked sweet potato and 1 cup mixed steamed broccoli and cauliflower, sprinkled with 1 teaspoon shredded Parmesan cheese.

For dessert: 1 cup sliced strawberries

410 calories, 33 grams protein, 40 grams carbohydrate,
14 grams fat, 10 grams fiber

Be Joyful

SONG OF THE DAY: "Wanna Be Starting Something" by Michael Jackson

Be Fit

WARM-UP: 3–5 minutes

CARDIO: 30–60 minutes

STRENGTH TRAINING: Killer Legs

STRETCH: 3–5 minutes

Killer Legs Workout

Squat and Cross Leg Lift

Stand with your feet hip-width apart. Squat with your arms bent forward at waist level (Position A). Contract your inner thigh muscles and lift your left leg across your body, extending your left arm to the side. Return to squatting position. Perform 15 reps, then repeat on the other side.

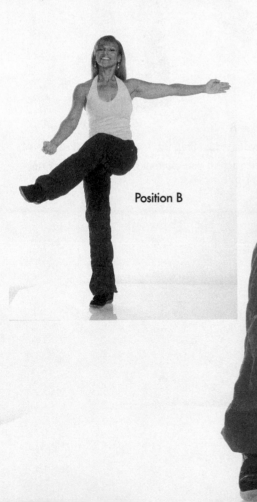

Position B

Position A

Back Lunge and Back Leg Lift

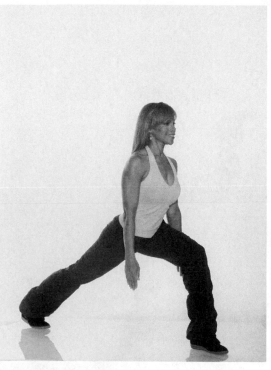

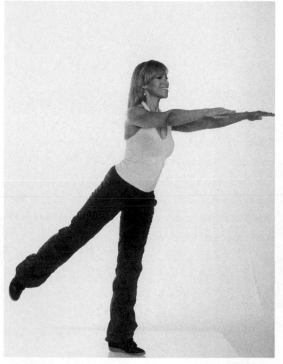

Position A

Position B

Stand with your feet slightly apart and your arms hanging by your sides. Step back into a lunge (Position A), then push off your back foot and lift your back leg up while contracting your buttocks and lifting your arms forward (Position B). Perform 15 reps, then repeat on the other side.

Single-Leg Dead Lift

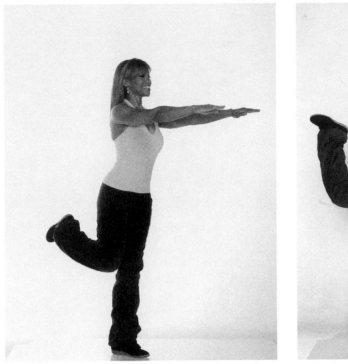 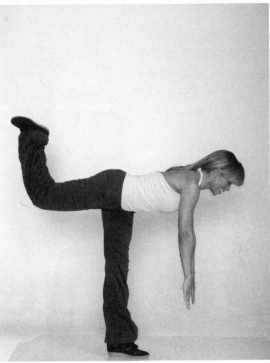

Position A

Position B

Stand on one leg with your other leg bent, your foot behind you, and your arms extended in front at shoulder level. Keep your back flat and bend at the hip until your back is parallel to the floor. Slowly return to standing position. Perform 15 reps, then switch legs and repeat.

Curtsy Lunge

Stand tall with feet slightly apart and hands in prayer position (Position A). Step diagonally back into a lunge with your left foot (Position B). Then bring your left foot forward and return to the starting position. Perform 15 reps, then switch to the other side and repeat.

REPEAT CIRCUIT 1–3 TIMES.

Position A

Position B

Be Faithful

*I beseech you therefore, brothers, by
the mercies of God, that you present your
bodies a living sacrifice, holy, acceptable to
God, which is your reasonable service.*

—ROMANS 12:1

Be Grateful

DORA'S STORY

*Donna's plan is inspirational and helps me get moving. The music is uplifting
and Donna is so encouraging. What I like best is that the program combines
workout and worship. Afterward I am thankful to be able to do the routine, and
I look forward to doing my next workout. I do the program five days a week, and
some days I also ride my bike through my neighborhood for thirty to forty-five
minutes.*

*In the past, sometimes I would get bored with working out. Usually within
about three months I was ready to move on to something else, but this program
is different. This time, I've stayed committed. I feel motivated and empowered to
focus on myself.*

*My diet is pretty good for the most part. I made a couple of changes, adding
more fruit, vegetables, and water. I eat a lot of fish, chicken, and beans for protein
and I rarely eat fried foods. I didn't need a big makeover for diet, but I definitely
needed to get in more exercise.*

*I go to school, I work, and I'm a caretaker, which means I have a lot on my
plate. I think the stress of not getting enough sleep and having a full schedule
contributed to my weight gain. In the past I felt overwhelmed and would slack
off from working out for a couple of months because I was taking care of my
responsibilities. Now I focus on taking care of myself and having more balance
in my life. I have more energy, I feel more productive, and I am now a size*

10! My goal is to lose 12 more pounds and drop another dress size. Donna is ushering a multitude of us into a lifestyle of fitness. Not a temporary fix, but a lifestyle.

With much joy,
Dora

Be Positive

Tomorrow is not promised, so seize the opportunity to live, love, and laugh. Every day, do something that brings you peace and joy.

Be Fruitful

BREAKFAST: Spinach, Mushroom, and Feta Scrambler with Orange

In a bowl, combine ½ cup thawed, drained spinach with ½ cup sliced mushrooms and set aside. In a nonstick skillet coated with cooking spray, scramble 1 whole egg and 2 additional egg whites. Add spinach and mushrooms. Cook through. Top with 1 ounce crumbled feta. Serve with 1 navel orange.

301 calories, 24 grams protein, 28 grams carbohydrate, 11 grams fat, 6 grams fiber

SNACK: Fruit and Cottage Cheese

⅓ cup low-fat (1% or 2%) cottage cheese, ½ navel orange, and 6 almonds.

144 calories, 10 grams protein, 15 grams carbohydrate, 5 grams fat, 3 grams fiber

LUNCH: Roast Turkey Cobb Salad

Combine 3 cups mixed salad greens with 3 ounces chopped, roasted, skinless turkey breast, 1 tablespoon crumbled blue cheese, 1 tablespoon bacon bits, ¼ sliced avocado, and ½ cup chopped tomato. Drizzle with approximately 2 tablespoons low-calorie ranch dressing. Serve with half a 6-inch whole-wheat pita pocket.

386 calories, 29 grams protein, 41 grams carbohydrate, 14 grams fat, 9 grams fiber

SNACK: Chocolate Almond Madness Smoothie

In a blender, combine 1 serving Chocolate Shakeology (or 6 ounces of any low-sugar protein powder), ¾ cup water, ¼ cup almond milk, ½ teaspoon almond extract, and 1 cup crushed ice.

> 157 calories, 17.5 grams protein, 19.5 grams carbohydrate,
> 1.5 grams fat, 3 grams fiber

DINNER: Beef Fajitas

Fill 1 warm whole-wheat tortilla (about 100 calories, or you may opt for two 50-calorie tortillas) with 3 ounces grilled flank steak cut into strips, 1 tablespoon low-fat grated cheddar cheese, ½ cup chopped tomatoes, and ¼ cup chopped white onion. Top with 2 tablespoons salsa. Serve with a mixed green salad and 1 tablespoon low-fat ranch dressing.

For dessert: sugar-free Jell-O with 1 tablespoon Cool Whip Lite

> 398 calories, 32 grams protein, 41 grams carbohydrate,
> 14 grams fat, 6 grams fiber

Be Joyful

SONG OF THE DAY: "Hey Ya" by OutKast

Be Fit

WARM-UP: 3–5 minutes
CARDIO: 30–60 minutes
STRENGTH TRAINING: Awesome Arms
STRETCH: 3–5 minutes

Awesome Arms Workout

Bent Row and Tricep Kickback

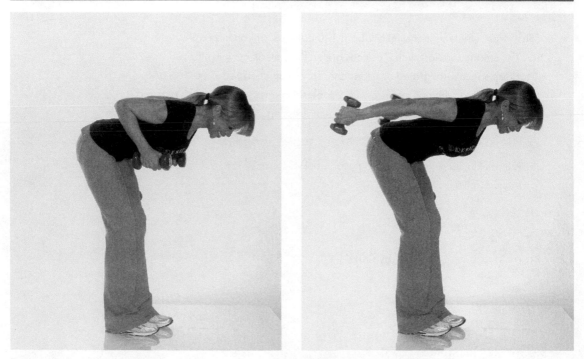

Position A

Position B

Stand with your feet shoulder-width apart and weights in your hands. Bend forward at your hips so that your back is parallel to the floor, keeping your abs tight. Raise your arms, bending them at the elbows, and contract your back muscles (Position A). Keeping your elbows close to your body, extend both arms back until they are parallel to the floor (Position B). Return to the starting position. Perform 15 reps.

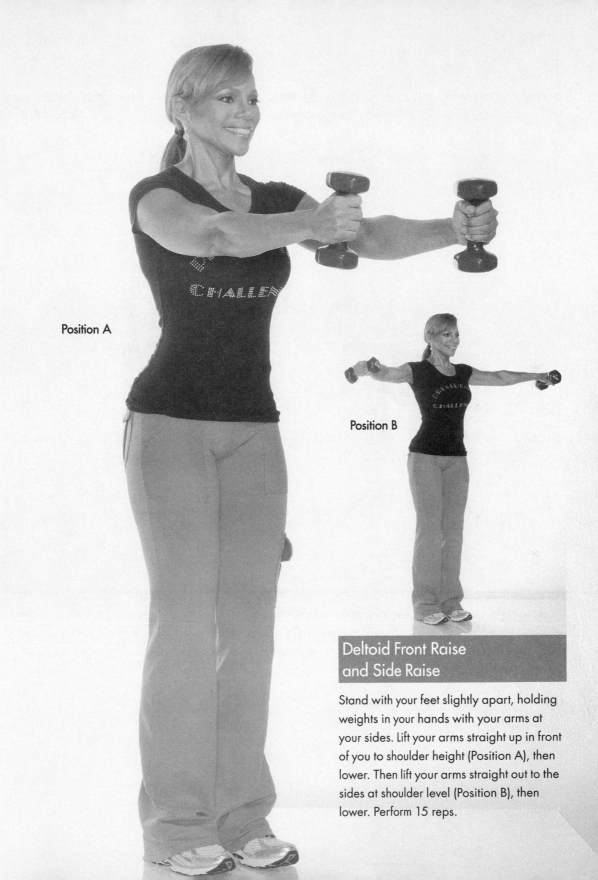

Position A

Position B

Deltoid Front Raise and Side Raise

Stand with your feet slightly apart, holding weights in your hands with your arms at your sides. Lift your arms straight up in front of you to shoulder height (Position A), then lower. Then lift your arms straight out to the sides at shoulder level (Position B), then lower. Perform 15 reps.

Dead Lift and Overhead Shoulder Press

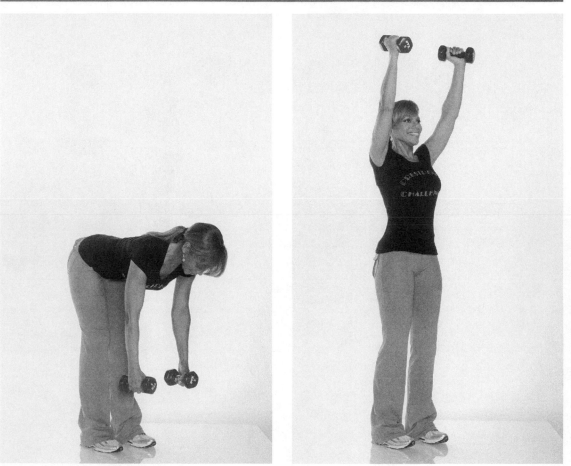

Position A   **Position B**

Stand with your feet shoulder-width apart, holding weights in your hands with your arms at your sides. Bend forward at the hip until your back is flat and parallel to the floor (Position A). Make sure you keep your abs contracted. Then lift up to a standing position and press the weights overhead, extending your arms (Position B). Return to the starting position. Perform 15 reps.

Bicep Curls

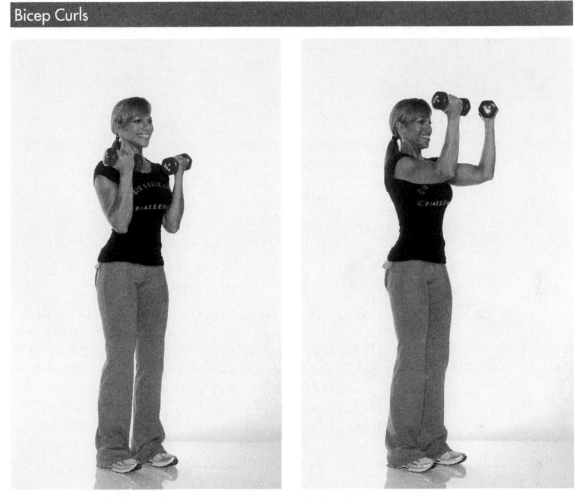

Position A   **Position B**

Stand with your feet slightly apart, holding weights and letting your arms hang by your sides. Curl the weights up to the front of your shoulders (Position A), then lift the elbows to chest level, raising the weights above your head (Position B). Lower the weights back to shoulder height, then return to the starting position. Perform 15 reps.

REPEAT CIRCUIT 1–3 TIMES.

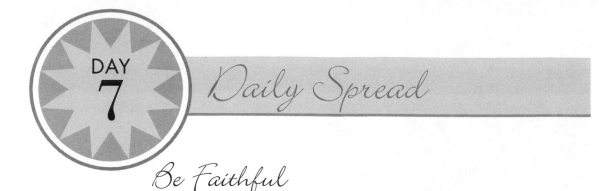

Be Faithful

Commit your way to the LORD; trust also in him;
and he shall bring it to pass.

—PSALM 37:5

Be Grateful

FRANK'S STORY

Frank Sanchez has been a part of the Boys and Girls Club most of his life. He became a member in 1969 at age six, when they opened a new club in the South Bronx. He had no idea that this would change his life forever. The club offered him the opportunity to develop as a young man, physically and socially, while laying the groundwork for him to become a leader with good character and integrity. His father worked long hours and didn't spend much time with him, but the club offered phenomenal male role models. Their Torch Club, which symbolizes the light of direction, taught him to be a leader. Later, in his teen years, he enrolled in the Keystone Club, which focuses on bringing people together with an emphasis on education, leadership, and community service.

At age fourteen, Frank was hired to teach kids baseball at the Boys and Girls Club, and for the last thirty-six years he has dedicated his life to teaching, nurturing, and empowering children. In addition, his mother ingrained in him the importance of helping kids. While he was growing up, his family adopted or sheltered many children, so although he had only two siblings, their home was always filled with lots of kids. His father, with whom he spent most of his time on weekends, taught Frank the value of hard work and of being a leader and a protector. Now Frank is teaching his sixteen-year-old son what was instilled in him. He lives in the spirit of helping children and knows he is fulfilling his God-given purpose.

Frank's job has taken him all over the world. For many years he worked with gang members as the senior director of delinquency prevention. He has worked with presidents and leaders as an advocate for children's rights. He is now the clubs' vice president of sports, entertainment, and alumni, and I have had the honor of working with him as a volunteer for the clubs for the past twenty years. Because of his passion and dedication, he is on track to transform lives of the next generation and to prepare our future leaders.

Be Positive

If you stay in neutral, nothing will change. Make the choice to embrace a shift in your health and in your life.

Be Fruitful

BREAKFAST: French Toast with Berries

Coat 2 slices of light-style wheat bread in a mixture of 1 whole egg beaten with 1 tablespoon skim milk. In a nonstick skillet coated with 1 teaspoon olive oil, sauté the coated bread until browned on both sides and cooked through. Top with ½ cup mixed berries and serve with ½ cup 1% cottage cheese.

> 304 calories, 25 grams protein, 29 grams carbohydrate, 11 grams fat, 5 grams fiber

SNACK: Turkey and Cheese

Serve 1 ounce deli turkey with 1 ounce soft goat cheese and ½ cup grapes.

> 157 calories, 11 grams protein, 14 grams carbohydrate, 6 grams fat, 1 gram fiber

LUNCH: Lemon-Dill Tuna Salad

In a large bowl, make a mixed green salad with 2 cups chopped romaine, ¼ chopped cucumber, 5 cherry tomatoes, and 1 chopped celery stalk. Top with 4 ounces drained water-packed tuna. Drizzle with dressing made from 2 teaspoons olive oil, 1 tablespoon lemon juice, and a sprinkle of dill (dry or fresh). Season with salt and pepper to taste. Serve with 2 pieces wheat melba toast and 1 sliced apple.

> 399 calories, 33 grams protein, 40 grams carbohydrate, 14 grams fat, 9 grams fiber

SNACK: Peanut Butter Apple

Serve 1 apple with 1 tablespoon peanut butter.

> 157 calories, 5 grams protein, 18 grams carbohydrate, 8 grams fat, 3 grams fiber

DINNER: Chicken and Vegetable Sauté

In a nonstick skillet coated with 2 teaspoons of olive oil, sauté 3 ounces cubed chicken breast, 1 cup cubed eggplant, ½ cup sliced red bell pepper, and ¼ cup sliced red onion. When vegetables are soft and chicken is cooked through, add 1 tablespoon teriyaki sauce, 1 tablespoon soy sauce, and any desired spices. Serve over ⅓ cup cooked brown rice (measured after cooking).

For dessert: 1 cup sliced strawberries with 1 teaspoon Cool Whip Lite

414 calories, 31 grams protein, 40 grams carbohydrate, 14 grams fat, 9 grams fiber

Be Joyful

SONG OF THE DAY: "Go Your Own Way" by Fleetwood Mac

Be Fit

Weekly Fitness Diary

_____

_____

_____

_____

_____

_____

_____

_____

_____

_____

_____

_____

_____

_____

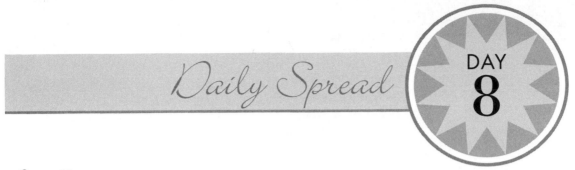

Be Faithful

Light in a messenger's eyes brings joy to the heart,
and good news gives health to the bones.

—PROVERBS 15:30

Be Grateful

CAROLYN'S STORY

Carolyn lost 45 lbs. in a four-month period.

My son Mike is a Body Gospel coach who has always encouraged me to keep going, work out, and live my best life. I am sixty-eight years old and have lost 45 pounds since I started the program. I was a little skeptical at first because I had no rhythm and I didn't think I could keep up with Donna. But when I watched her tape, Pam, who does the modified version of the workout on the DVDs, became my new best friend, and Donna's encouragement and warm spirit kept me motivated and moving. Her magical voice was so inviting that I felt like we were girlfriends working out together. Donna is beautiful inside and out, and her infectious energy keeps me pumped up!

Part of my inspiration was hearing my thirteen-year-old granddaughter say, "Grandma, we are going to do this together!" We worked out with the videos and went to the playground. We played "monkey in the middle" and enjoyed going down the slide. My granddaughter became my workout buddy and a source of inspiration. There is no way I am going to stop with the best support system ever—my granddaughter, my son, and Donna pushing me and helping me every step of the way. Some of the most inspiring words came from my granddaughter: "You look beautiful, and your age must be going backwards."

Sincerely,
Carolyn

Be Positive

Keep taking steps toward a better body and life. Inhale positive thoughts and exhale negative thoughts.

Be Fruitful

BREAKFAST: Scrambled Eggs and Turkey Bacon

In a nonstick skillet coated with cooking spray, scramble 3 egg whites. Add 1 ounce reduced-fat cheddar cheese. Serve with 2 slices turkey bacon, 1 slice light-style wheat bread, and 1 cup cubed melon.

298 calories, 27 grams protein, 28 grams carbohydrate, 10 grams fat, 4 grams fiber

SNACK: Open-Faced Turkey Sandwich

Serve 1 slice wheat toast topped with 1½ ounces sliced white-meat turkey and ⅛ sliced avocado.

164 calories, 11 grams protein, 15 grams carbohydrate, 7 grams fat, 4 grams fiber

LUNCH: Roast Beef and Goat Cheese Wrap

Spread 1 ounce soft goat cheese on a whole-wheat wrap (about 100 calories). Layer 2 ounces lean roast beef with ¼ cup shredded romaine lettuce, ¼ cup alfalfa sprouts, ¼ red bell pepper, sliced, and 3 cucumber slices; roll and cut in half. Serve with a small mandarin orange.

397 calories, 30 grams protein, 40 grams carbohydrate, 15 grams fat, 6 grams fiber

SNACK: Blueberry Almond Yogurt

Combine ½ cup low-fat plain yogurt with 1 tablespoon slivered almonds and ⅓ cup fresh or frozen blueberries. Add no- or low-calorie sweetener (Stevia) if desired.

153 calories, 8 grams protein, 15 grams carbohydrate, 6 grams fat, 1.5 grams fiber

DINNER: Asian Chicken Salad

In a shallow dish, marinate a 3-ounce chicken breast in teriyaki sauce for approximately 10 minutes. Coat nonstick skillet with cooking spray and sauté chicken until done. Cover and set aside. In a large salad bowl, toss together 2 cups shredded mixed greens, 1 cup shredded napa cabbage, 1 tablespoon slivered almonds, 1 shredded carrot, and ½ cup drained canned mandarin oranges. Add warm chicken to salad, then toss with 2 tablespoons light-style sesame dressing. Garnish with 4 crumbled baked tortilla chips. Season with salt and pepper to taste.

For dessert: 1 cup sugar-free Jell-O with 1 teaspoon Cool Whip Lite

409 calories, 32 grams protein, 37 grams carbohydrate,
14 grams fat, 9 grams fiber

Be Joyful

SONG OF THE DAY: "Karma Chameleon" by Culture Club

Be Fit

WARM-UP: 3–4 minutes
CARDIO AND STRENGTH TRAINING: Playground Boot Camp
STRETCH: 3–5 minutes

Playground Boot Camp Workout

Hula-Hoop

Exercise 1

Step into a Hula-hoop with your feet wide apart and your knees slightly bent. Pull the Hula-hoop up to your waist and give it a spin. Keep it moving by circling your hips around and around. Perform for 1 minute.

Incline Push-Ups

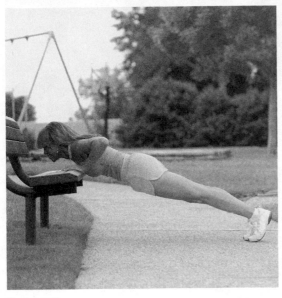

Exercise 2

Find a bench at the playground. Lean forward, place your hands on the bench, and back your feet up until you are in push-up position. Keep your abs tightened and your body in a straight line. Bend your elbows, lowering your chest to the bench, and then straighten your arms back to the starting position. Repeat for 1 minute.

Jumping Jacks

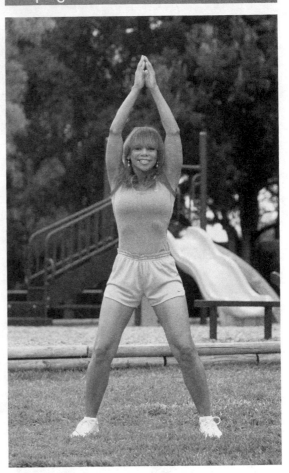

Exercise 3

Stand tall with your feet together and your arms alongside your body. Jump your feet apart as you raise your arms above your head. Return to the starting position. Perform for 1 minute.

Step-Ups

Exercise 4
Stand in front of a bench and step up onto it. Then step back down. Repeat for 30 seconds with your right foot leading and then for another 30 seconds with your left foot leading.

Jump Rope

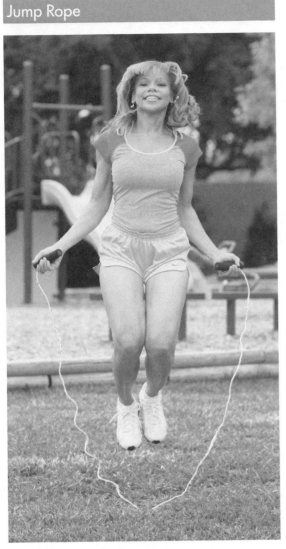

Hanging Knee Lifts

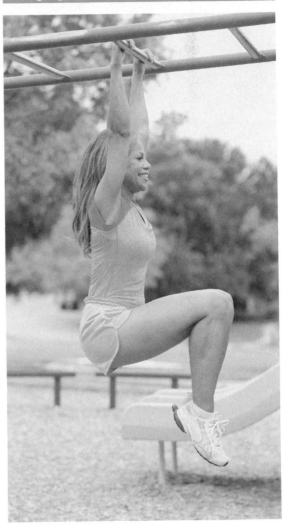

Exercise 5

With or without a rope, start jumping, hopping either from one foot to the other or with both feet together. Perform for 1 minute.

Exercise 6

Grab hold of some monkey bars with your hands shoulder-width apart and palms facing forward. (Your legs can be straight or slightly bent.) Contract your abs and pull your knees up to your rib cage. Straighten your legs and repeat. Perform for 1 minute.

Bench Hops

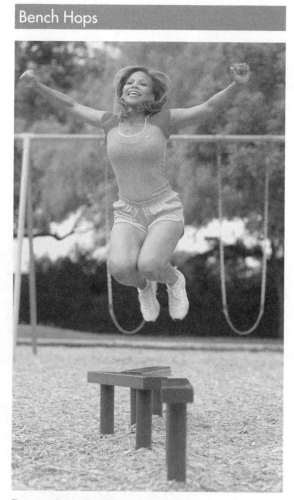

Exercise 7

Find a bench without a back, or find a short, narrow wall. Stand to one side of the bench and hop over it. Repeat from the other side. Perform for 1 minute.

Crab Crawl

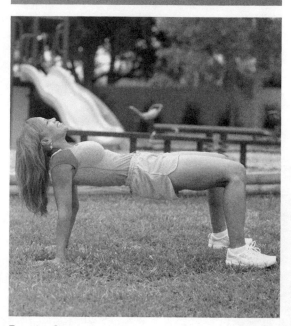

Exercise 8

Get down on your hands and feet on the ground or grass, front side up and with your abs contracted. Step forward with one foot and hand, then bring the other foot and hand forward the same distance. Lead on one side for 30 seconds, lead on the other for 30 seconds.

REPEAT CIRCUIT 2–3 TIMES.

Be Faithful

You shall also decree a thing, and it shall be established
to you: and the light shall shine on your ways.

—JOB 22:28

Be Grateful

PAT'S STORY

Alzheimer's is a kind of dementia that causes problems with cognitive ability,
behavior, and memory loss. My dad has dementia, but with love, care, and
family, he is doing pretty darn good. For instance, he remembers who owes
him money and all the beautiful women he hit on in church. Like my dad, Pat
Summitt has Alzheimer's but has taken a positive approach and is not allowing
this disease to get the best of her. Instead, she has chosen to overcome this disease.

Pat Summitt knows all too well how to defeat the odds. She started coaching
at the University of Tennessee at the tender age of twenty-two during a time
when women had no voice. She was barely older than her players, but that did
not stop her. Pat won eight national titles and 1,098 games, which is more than
any other major basketball coach, man or woman. In her early coaching career,
she was given a budget of only $250 a month. She washed the girls' uniforms
herself because they only had one set. She and the players had to sleep on mats in
the opponents' gym because she could not afford a hotel. Like my dad, Pat has a
strong spirit, and she has a will to live.

Pat has taught her teams discipline, determination, and humility. She
emphasizes that hard work pays off. Staying strong in body helps her stay
strong in mind and spirit. She will need to apply these same principles to fight
Alzheimer's, this incurable disease. Those who live with dementia, like my dad
and Pat, must continue to exercise their minds and their bodies so that they can
continue to live productive lives.

Be Positive

Every day, be grateful and write down at least
one thing you are thankful for.

Be Fruitful

BREAKFAST: Cottage Cheese and Fruit Parfait

In a tall glass, layer ⅔ cup of 1% cottage cheese with ½ cup sliced
strawberries, ½ cup cubed apple, ⅓ cup high-fiber breakfast cereal, and
1 tablespoon crushed walnuts. Sprinkle with 1 teaspoon cinnamon and
1 packet of sweetener (Splenda or Stevia) if desired.

> 295 calories, 24 grams protein, 30 grams carbohydrate,
> 11 grams fat, 5 grams fiber

SNACK: Ham and Cheese

Arrange 1 ounce ham with 1 ounce low-fat cheddar on 3 pieces whole-wheat
melba toast.

> 157 calories, 12 grams protein, 16 grams carbohydrate,
> 4 grams fat, 1.5 grams fiber

LUNCH: Classic Chicken Salad Wrap

In a bowl, combine 3 ounces chopped grilled chicken breast, 1 tablespoon
reduced-fat mayonnaise, and 1 chopped celery stalk. Season with salt and
pepper to taste. Spread chicken salad on 6-inch whole-wheat wrap (about
100 calories). Layer with slices of red onion and roll up. Serve with ⅓ cup plain
nonfat yogurt topped with 1 tablespoon chopped walnuts.

> 388 calories, 34 grams protein, 40 grams carbohydrate,
> 13 grams fat, 4 grams fiber

SNACK: Frozen Daiquiri Smoothie

In a blender, combine 1 serving Greenberry Shakeology (or 6 ounces of any
low-sugar protein powder), ½ teaspoon coconut extract, ¼ cup pineapple,
1 cup water, and ½ cup ice (add more for additional thickness).

> 158 calories, 17 grams protein, 22 grams carbohydrate,
> 1 gram fat, 3 grams fiber

DINNER: Sliced Flank Steak

Broil a 3-ounce flank steak for approximately 6 minutes on each side, or until done. Slice and top with 1 cup mushrooms and onions sautéed in 1 teaspoon olive oil. Serve with 10 steamed asparagus spears and ½ medium baked potato.

For dessert: ½ pink grapefruit, cut in quarters

404 calories, 32 grams protein, 41 grams carbohydrate, 14 grams fat, 6 grams fiber

Be Joyful

SONG OF THE DAY: "Livin' la Vida Loca" by Ricky Martin

Be Fit

WARM-UP: 3–5 minutes

POWER PLAY STRENGTH-TRAINING CARDIO: 30–60 minutes

STRETCH: 3–5 minutes

Power Play Workout

Squat and Thrust

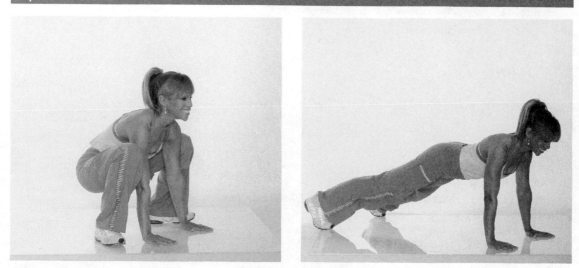

Position A

Position B

Stand tall with your arms alongside your body and your abs contracted, then squat down and place your hands on the floor inside your feet (Position A). Thrust your feet to a push-up position (Position B), then jump back to a squat. Return to the starting position. Repeat for 2 minutes.

Mountain Climber

Squat and place your hands on the floor. Walk your feet out so your legs are straight, and contract your abs (Position A). Lift one knee up to your chest and touch your toe to the floor (Position B), then return to the starting position. Repeat on the other side. Alternate for 2 minutes.

Position A

Position B

Lunge and Front Kick

Stand tall with your feet slightly apart and your arms bent in front of your chest. Step back into a lunge with your right foot (Position A). Push off your right foot and perform a front kick (Position B). Repeat for 1 minute. Switch sides and continue for 1 minute.

Position A

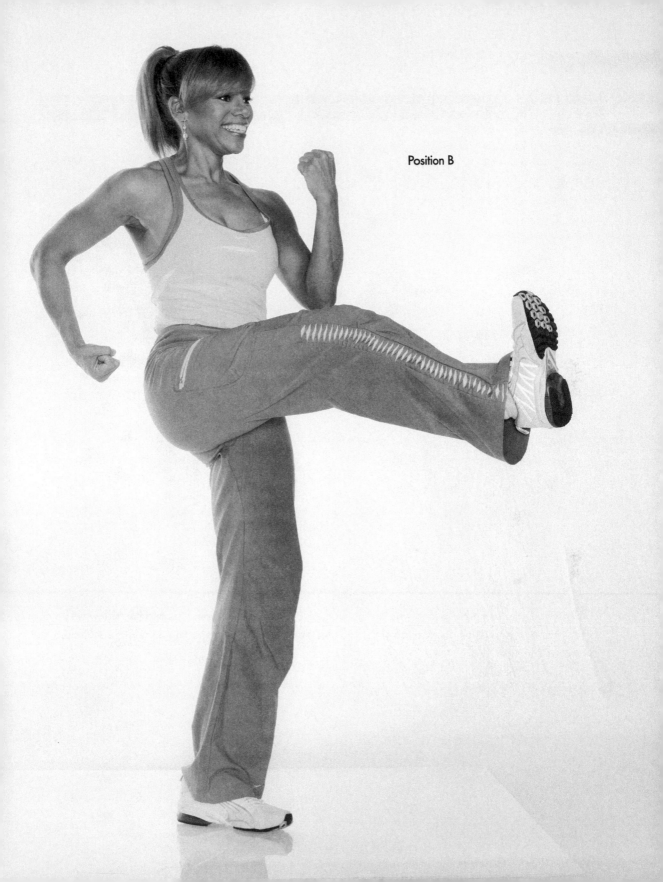

Position B

Skater

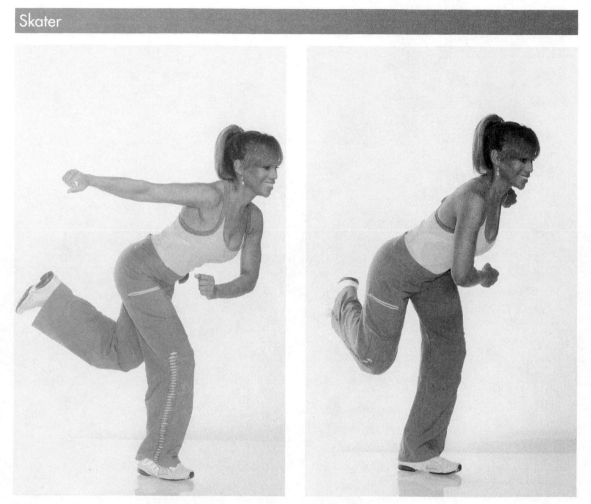

Position A   Position B

Stand tall with your feet together and your abs contracted. Bend forward at your hips and hop sideways from one foot to the other, putting one arm in front of you and the other behind, alternating arms with each hop. Perform for 2 minutes.

REPEAT CIRCUIT 3–5 TIMES.

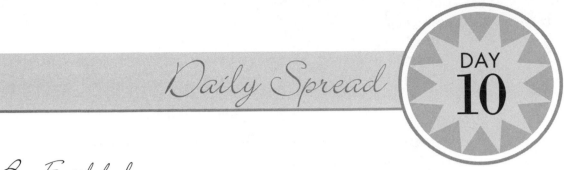

Be Faithful

*Iron sharpens iron; so a man sharpens
the countenance of his friend.*

—PROVERBS 27:17

Be Grateful

REECIE'S STORY

Reecie weighed 390 lbs. at her heaviest and lost 90 lbs. in ten months.

From the time I was about three years old, I was as wide as I was tall. I always struggled with being overweight. Finally one day I called Donna and told her, "I have made up my mind; I can do it this time." Donna asked me to do a half marathon to help me lose weight and keep up a can-do attitude. I was excited at first, but then it hit me. I said to myself, a half marathon—that's 13.1 miles! I started training, but then all kinds of craziness happened in my life. I didn't know if I could finish the race, and some of my friends and family doubted me. But Donna was always positive. She said, "You can do this—just stay focused and believe in yourself."

The morning of the race, I prayed, "Okay, God, whatever your will is, let your will be done." I put on my iPod, and my friend and I started the race. We were doing fine, but we took such a long time that after a while the race's cones disappeared. I guess one can say we were lost. We walked an additional three miles. We called Donna on the phone. She said, "Where the hell are you all? I'm just kidding." Donna and Tarra, the director of Body Gospel—my spiritual angels—prayed with me and guided us to the finish line.

If you believe, nothing is impossible. When Donna put the medal on me after we crossed the finish line, I was overwhelmed with joy and a sense of accomplishment. Donna challenged me to reach beyond what I could see. It means so much now to know that whatever I set my mind to, I can do. There are no more excuses. I don't have to settle for less than what I want or less than what I deserve.

   Love,
   Reecie

P.S. I have lost 90 pounds, and I am on track to achieving my goal of losing 110 more pounds.

Be Positive

Plan your day wisely so that you set yourself up for success. Preparation, planning, and execution are the keys to success!

Be Fruitful

BREAKFAST: Chicken Sausage and Egg White Burrito

Scramble 4 egg whites or ½ cup egg substitute in a nonstick skillet coated with cooking spray. Layer one 6-inch whole-wheat tortilla with the scrambled eggs and 2 cooked, chopped chicken sausage links (about 60 calories each, or 120 to 130 calories total). Top with 2 tablespoons salsa and roll up.

   297 calories, 25 grams protein, 28 grams carbohydrate,
   11 grams fat, 2.5 grams fiber

SNACK: Crunchy Fruit Yogurt

Combine ½ cup low-fat plain yogurt with 1 tablespoon chopped walnuts and ½ cup cubed cantaloupe.

   152 calories, 9 grams protein, 16 grams carbohydrate,
   6 grams fat, 1 gram fiber

LUNCH: Caesar Salad with Grilled Shrimp

In a large bowl, toss a salad of prewashed romaine salad greens with low-fat Caesar dressing. Top with 3 ounces herb-grilled shrimp. Sprinkle with 2 tablespoons grated Parmesan cheese and ½ cup croutons, whole-wheat if possible (about 120 to 140 calories for the ½ cup portion). Finish with a cup of mixed berries, fresh or frozen.

   410 calories, 31 grams protein, 40 grams carbohydrate,
   13 grams fat, 6 grams fiber

SNACK: Vanilla Almond Berry Smoothie

In a blender, combine 1 scoop Greenberry Shakeology (or 6 ounces of any low-sugar protein powder), ¼ cup vanilla-flavored almond milk, ¾ cup water, ½ teaspoon vanilla extract, and 1 cup ice (add more for desired thickness).

157 calories, 17.5 grams protein, 19.5 grams carbohydrate,
1.5 grams fat, 3 grams fiber

DINNER: Marinated Pork Chop

Marinate a 3-ounce lean center-cut pork chop in low-calorie teriyaki sauce or another low-calorie bottled marinade. Broil on both sides until cooked through. Sauté 1 teaspoon sesame seeds in nonstick cooking spray, then add to 1 cup fresh baby spinach. Serve the pork chop on a bed of fresh spinach and sesame seeds, along with a baked potato.

For dessert: ½ cup unsweetened applesauce

404 calories, 28 grams protein, 40 grams carbohydrate,
12 grams fat, 5 grams fiber

Be Joyful

SONG OF THE DAY: "Love Train" by the O'Jays

Be Fit

WARM-UP: 3–5 minutes
CARDIO: 30–60 minutes
STRENGTH TRAINING: Ablicious
STRETCH: 3–5 minutes

Ablicious Workout

Knee Tuck and Leg Extensions

Sit on the floor or a mat with your hands behind your buttocks and elbows slightly bent. Bend your legs and bring your knees toward your chest, lifting your feet off the mat (Position A). Lean back and extend your legs (Position B), then return to bent knees in front of chest. Perform 15–20 reps.

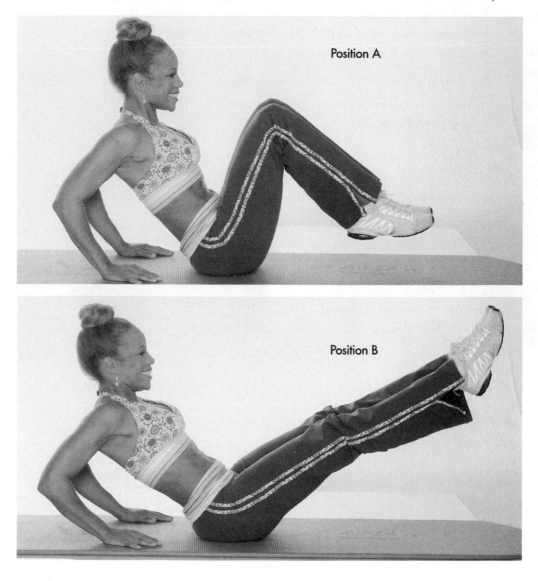

Position A

Position B

Scissors

Lie on your back, with one arm above your head, resting on the floor. Tighten your abs, curl up until your shoulders start to lift off the floor. Lift one leg up, reaching for it with the opposite arm (Position A). Switch legs and repeat to complete one set (Position B). Perform 15–20 reps.

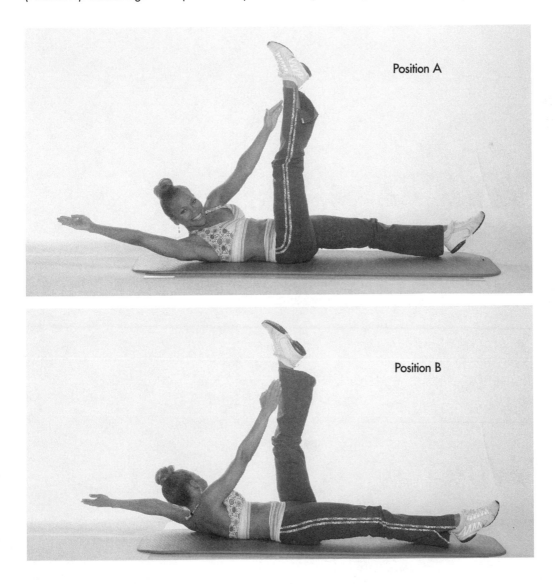

Position A

Position B

Hundreds

Lie on your back with your legs extended at a 45-degree angle and your arms resting on the floor with your palms down (Position A). Inhale and pull your navel toward the floor. Exhale and lift your head and shoulders up while keeping your lower back on the floor. Lift your arms slightly off the floor and pulse up and down (Position B). Repeat for 10 exhales and 10 inhales. Lower your feet to the floor, then lower your head to the floor.

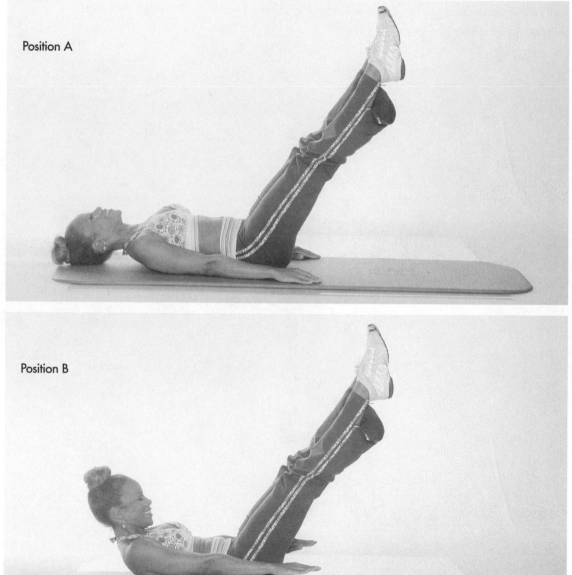

Position A

Position B

Boxer's Curl

Lie on your back, elbows out to the sides, knees bent, and feet flat on the floor. Contract your abs, lift your shoulders off the floor, and clench your hands into boxing position. Rotate your torso to one side while extending the opposite arm across your body (Position A). Rotate back to the center, keeping your shoulders off the floor. Bend at the elbows and bring your bent arms and clenched fists back to your sides. Rotate to the opposite side while extending your arm across your body (Position B) to complete one rep. Perform 15–20 reps.

REPEAT CIRCUIT 1–3 TIMES.

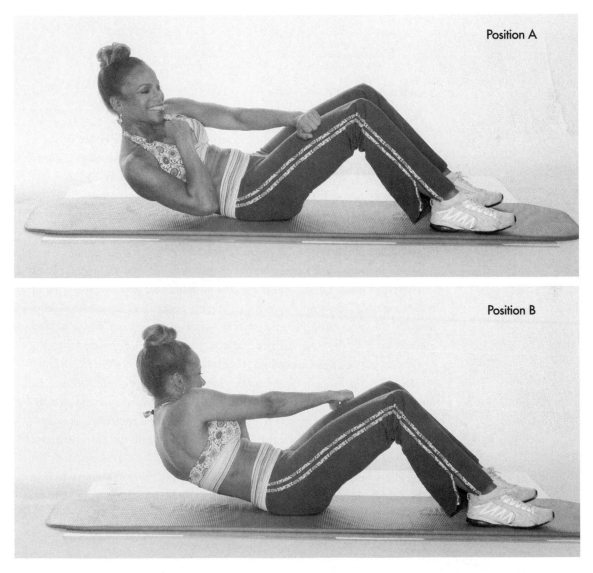

Position A

Position B

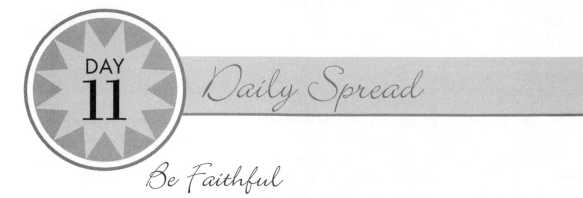

Be Faithful

Therefore, if anyone is in Christ, he is a new creation;
the old has gone, the new has come!
—2 CORINTHIANS 5:17

Be Grateful

TARRA'S STORY

One of my most fulfilling achievements was being ranked number one as a pharmaceutical sales rep in my district and one of the top in the nation. The job was challenging, yet fulfilling. I had the opportunity to come face-to-face with physicians and provide them with current and accurate information about a variety of drugs. But being in the health care industry, my spirit was grieved from seeing many people suffering.

One day my manager called to advise me that seven hundred employees would lose their jobs nationwide, including me. I was told that October 8 would be my last day. As a mother of six children with a husband who was unemployed and bills piling up, I should have been shaking in my boots. But in my heart, I felt that God had opened the door for me to minister on my job, and that if he was allowing that door to close, then he had a bigger door opening for me.

On October 8, I went into prayer. God told me not to worry but to celebrate the date. He said, "October is the tenth month, and ten represents a whole." He said the number 8 represented new beginnings. He said, "I am giving you a whole new beginning. I am taking you to places you have never been. Your eyes have not seen, your ears have not heard, neither has entered into the hearts of man the things that I have in store for you."

A call came in from my friend Donna Richardson Joyner as she was leaving Paris. God laid me on her heart to help launch Body Gospel. She didn't know that I was unemployed. Tears rolled down my face when I got off the phone. God had spoken to Donna about me, and she obeyed his voice to hire me. I flew to Los

Angeles to meet Donna and the rest is history. I am currently the director of Body Gospel. I travel around the world with Donna, helping people to live healthier, happier lives. One day we might be in a church in the 'hood and the next at the White House. Only God could give me "a whole new beginning" and take me to places I had never been. He used Donna as a vehicle for me to continue to minister all for his glory!

    Tarra

Be Positive

Move to improve. Take steps to be physically active daily. You know the saying: "If you don't move it, you lose it."

Be Fruitful

BREAKFAST: Breakfast Stack

On half a whole-wheat English muffin, layer ½ cup steamed spinach, 2 slices pan-grilled Canadian bacon, 1 egg (fried sunny-side up or over in a nonstick skillet coated with cooking spray), and 1 slice tomato. Serve with ½ cup cantaloupe.

> 289 calories, 24 grams protein, 28 grams carbohydrate, 10 grams fat, 6 grams fiber

SNACK: Berry Ricotta

Mix ⅓ cup part-skim ricotta cheese with ½ cup fresh or frozen blueberries or strawberries and 1 teaspoon slivered almonds. Sprinkle with cinnamon; add sweetener if desired.

> 159 calories, 10 grams protein, 15 grams carbohydrate, 6 grams fat, 1 gram fiber

LUNCH: Curry Chicken Salad with Mixed Greens

In a bowl, combine 3 ounces chopped poached chicken breast, 1 chopped celery stalk, ½ chopped green apple, 2 tablespoons dried cranberries, 1 tablespoon low-fat mayonnaise, and ¼ teaspoon curry powder (add more curry if desired). Mix and scoop onto a bed of mixed greens. Sprinkle with 1 tablespoon chopped walnuts. Serve with a small whole-grain dinner roll.

> 411 calories, 31 grams protein, 39 grams carbohydrate, 15 grams fat, 5 grams fiber

SNACK: Sliced Apple and Turkey

Serve 1½ ounces deli turkey breast with ½ small apple, sliced, and 10 unsalted almonds.

150 calories, 11 grams protein, 15 grams carbohydrate,
6 grams fat, 3 grams fiber

DINNER: Shrimp and Veggie Stir-Fry

In a nonstick skillet over medium-high heat, add 1 tablespoon olive oil and sauté 4 ounces cleaned large shrimp, ¼ cup chopped red onion, and 1 cup broccoli florets. When shrimp is cooked through and veggies are soft (approximately 8 to 10 minutes), add 1 tablespoon soy sauce, 1 tablespoon low-calorie teriyaki sauce, and any desired spices. Serve with ½ cup cooked whole-wheat couscous.

For dessert: 1 cup cantaloupe, cubed

390 calories, 30 grams protein, 41 grams carbohydrate,
12 grams fat, 5 grams fiber

Be Joyful

SONG OF THE DAY: "Moves Like Jagger" by Maroon 5

Be Fit

WARM-UP: 3–5 minutes
CARDIO: 30–60 minutes
STRENGTH TRAINING: Body Beautiful
STRETCH: 3–5 minutes

Body Beautiful Workout

Decline Bench Press and Leg Lift

Lie on your back, holding weights in your hands with your elbows out to the sides, your knees bent, and your feet flat on the ground (Position A). Contract your buttocks, lift your hips, and extend one leg. At the same time, press the weights toward the ceiling (Position B). Then lower your hips, leg, and arms to the floor. Repeat on the opposite side. Perform 15 reps.

Position A

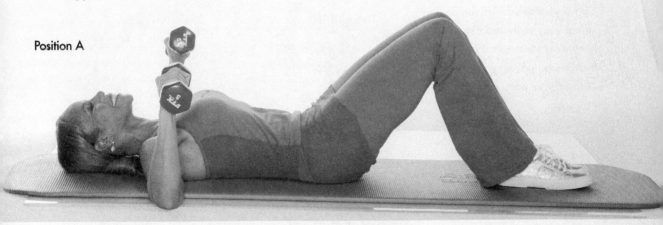

Position B

Calf Raise and Tricep Extension

Stand with your feet slightly apart, your arms bent above, and your hands holding weights behind your head (Position A). Roll up through the balls of your feet, lifting your heels off the floor and extending your arms straight above your head (Position B). Lower your heels and bend your arms down to the start position. Remember to keep your elbows close to your ears. Perform 15 reps.

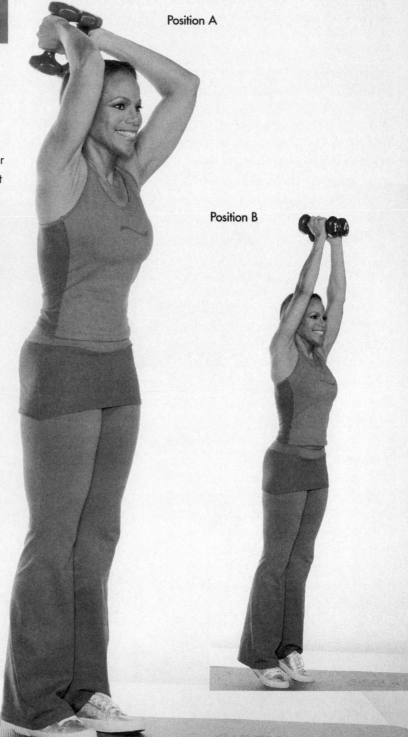

Position A

Position B

Push-Up Side Plank

Lie facedown on the floor with your hands flat and your elbows bent. Lift your body to a low push-up with your elbows bent (Position A). Keep your abs tight and your body straight, and press up by straightening your arms. Transfer your weight onto one hand and extend the opposite hand toward the ceiling (Position B). Return to the low push-up position, then repeat on the other side. Perform 10–15 reps.

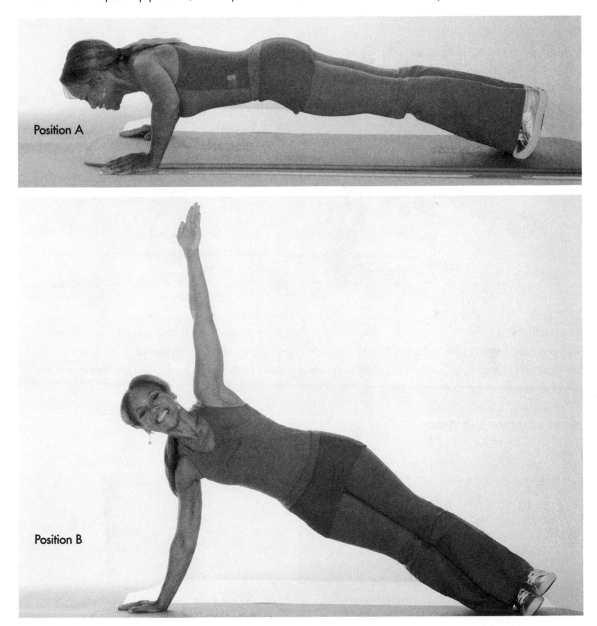

Position A

Position B

Front Lunge and Bicep Curl

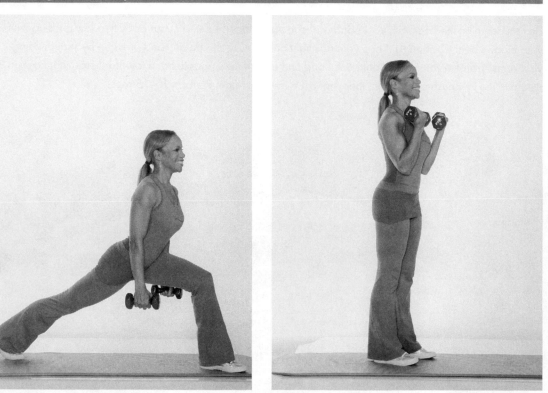

Position A   **Position B**

Stand tall with your feet slightly apart, weights in your hands, and your arms by your sides. Lunge forward with one foot, bending the knee (Position A). Return to a standing position, lifting the weights toward your shoulders and keeping your elbows tight by your sides (Position B). Return to the starting position and repeat with the opposite foot. Perform 15 reps.

REPEAT CIRCUIT 1–3 TIMES.

Be Faithful

*Whether therefore you eat, or drink, or whatever
you do, do all to the glory of God.*

—1 CORINTHIANS 10:31

Be Grateful

MOM'S STORY

My mom is seventy-two years young, and she is faithfully fit and fabulous!
I hope what she has is in our genes, because she lives her life with zest and zeal!
She is a social butterfly, the life of the party. She can dance circles around my
friends and me, and she has her own signature moves. I tell her that one day she
is going to do her "cute dip" (a squat with fingers pointed out) and not be able to
get back up again. She says, "I will do it until I can't do it anymore."

At one time, my mother had some health concerns, but she faced her
challenges head-on. Not only did she become healthier, but she even started a
fitness and health ministry at her church. She would always say, "Donna, we
need a workout that has some good gospel and Christian music."

My mom and other members of her church would follow my old workout
videos with the volume down, then play gospel music and get their praise on.
When I finally created the faith and fitness programs and went out on tour,
my mom was right there at my side. She is still the best cheerleader I have,
not because I'm her baby girl but because she has witnessed family, friends,
and church members change their lives to combat illness and break unhealthy
habits.

My mom exemplifies strength, wisdom, kindness, grace, and beauty! I pray
that I can do all that she is doing at her age, and then some.

Be Positive

Fuel your body with good nutrition so that it can perform at its best. Remember, you are what you eat.

Be Fruitful

BREAKFAST: Veggie Omelet with Grapefruit

In a nonstick skillet coated with 1 teaspoon olive oil, make an omelet with 1 whole egg, 3 egg whites, 3 chopped white mushrooms, ½ cup spinach, and ¼ cup chopped onion. Serve with 1 fresh grapefruit.

> 307 calories, 25 grams protein, 31 grams carbohydrate, 10 grams fat, 6 grams fiber

SNACK: Fruit and Cheese Plate

1 small pear and 1 ounce reduced-fat cheddar cheese.

> 150 calories, 10 grams protein, 17 grams carbohydrate, 5 grams fat, 3 grams fiber

LUNCH: South of the Border Burger

Form 4 ounces lean turkey into a patty and broil for 5 minutes on each side. Place burger in a whole-grain hamburger bun and top with ¼ cup black beans, 2 slices tomato, and 1 to 2 tablespoons salsa. Serve with a small mixed green salad tossed with 1 tablespoon low-calorie salad dressing.

> 385 calories, 30 grams protein, 39 grams carbohydrate, 13 grams fat, 8 grams fiber

SNACK: Tuna and Crackers

Mix 2 ounces tuna with 1 teaspoon light mayonnaise and 1 teaspoon lemon juice. Serve on 5 whole-wheat crackers (crackers should total about 50 calories).

> 158 calories, 11 grams protein, 16 grams carbohydrate, 6 grams fat, 5 grams fiber

DINNER: Healthy Chicken Parmesan

Place a 3-ounce grilled chicken breast in a baking pan and top with ⅓ cup tomato sauce. Cover with 1 ounce shredded part-skim mozzarella cheese and bake until bubbly. Serve with 1 cup steamed spinach and a mixed green salad dressed with 2 tablespoons light Italian dressing (approximately 40 calories per 2 tablespoons).

For dessert: ½ cup fresh or frozen berries

389 calories, 34 grams protein, 41 grams carbohydrate,
11 grams fat, 9 grams fiber

Be Joyful

SONG OF THE DAY: "Thankful" by Mary Mary

Be Fit

WARM-UP: 3–5 minutes
CARDIO: Body Gospel
STRENGTH TRAINING: 10–20 minutes
STRETCH: 3–5 minutes

Body Gospel Workout

Side-to-Side Celebration

Exercise 1

Start with your feet together and your arms at your sides. Step to one side, shifting your weight to that foot while you open your hands wide with your palms facing forward. Return to the starting position with both feet together. Perform for 2 minutes, alternating sides.

Praise Lunge

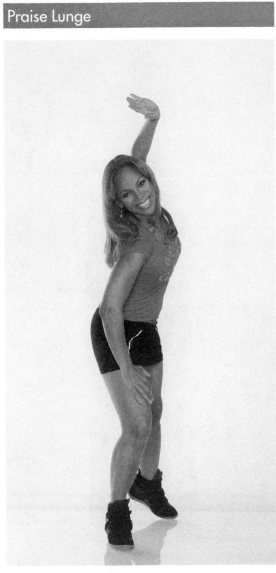

Glorious Jumping Jack

Exercise 2

Stand tall with your feet together and your arms at your sides. Step forward into a lunge with one leg while swinging the opposite arm behind you. Return to the starting position and repeat on the other side. Alternate sides and perform for 2 minutes.

Exercise 3

Stand tall with your feet together and your arms at your sides. Jump out, lifting your arms above your head and your chest to the heavens. Return to the starting position. Perform for 2 minutes.

Happy Hop

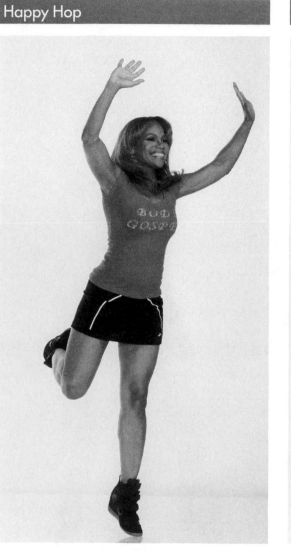

Joyful Run

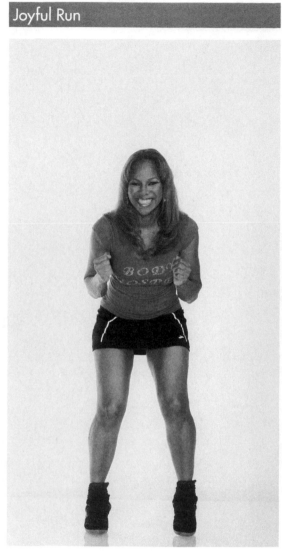

Exercise 4

Stand tall with your feet slightly apart and your arms hanging by your sides. Double-hop onto your left foot, double-pumping your arms. Double-hop onto your right foot and double-pump your arms. Alternate from side to side. Perform for 2 minutes.

Exercise 5

Stand straight with your feet shoulder-width apart. Bend at your hips, lowering your body into a squat position. Start a quick run in place, keeping your weight on the balls of your feet. Run in place for 2 minutes.

Hallelujah Knee Lifts

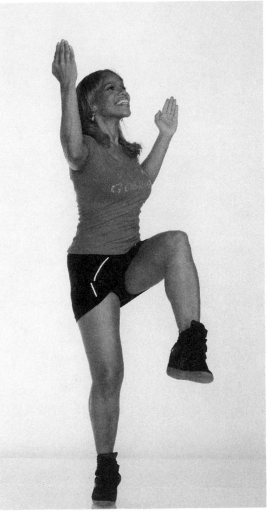

Punching-Bag Victory

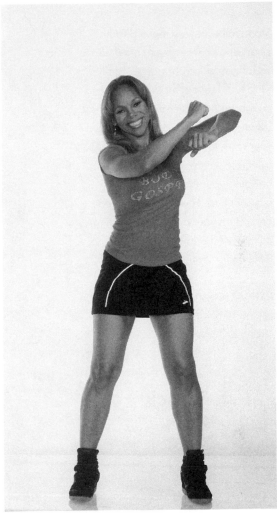

Exercise 6

Stand tall with your feet slightly apart, your arms hanging to the sides. Lift your left knee up and bend your arms to shoulder level while twisting to the left. Return to the start position, then repeat on the other side. Alternate sides and perform for 2 minutes.

Exercise 7

Stand with your feet slightly more than shoulder-width apart and bend your knees. Lift your arms and imitate punching a speed bag. Punch for 8 counts on the right, then repeat on the left. Perform for 2 minutes.

Super Kicks

Exercise 8

Stand tall with your feet hip-width apart and your arms extended above your head with your palms together. Kick your left foot forward and bend your arms down in front of your chest. Lower your left foot down and return your arms to the starting position. Do a front kick with your right foot forward, bringing your arms down in front of your chest. Lower your right foot and return your arms to the starting position. Alternate from side to side. Perform for 2 minutes.

REPEAT CIRCUIT 2–3 TIMES.

Be Faithful

Have I not commanded you? Be strong and courageous.
Do not be afraid; do not be discouraged, for the Lord
your God will be with you wherever you go.
—JOSHUA 1:9

Be Grateful

ROXANNE'S STORY

Roxanne weighed 154 lbs. when she began and has lost 39 lbs.

One day a church member told me about a faith-based weight-loss program that was about to kick off at the gym where she worked. As the first lady of a church, I was totally excited because I had never heard of this kind of program. I spoke to my husband, and we agreed to participate together. We knew that we had to do something different with regard to our health.

A few months earlier I had made a decision to take better care of myself so that I could meet the demands of being a wife, soccer mom, and choir director, as well as wearing several other hats at our church. I led by example, and my husband followed suit. The first few sessions with Donna were difficult because they were held in the morning and I am not a morning person. However, every time I went I was inspired, and I began to look forward to the next session.

When you work out with Christian or gospel music, it's like worship; your soul is stirred up. The music ministers to me, and I love how the class ends with prayer and scripture. As a Christian, it is God's word that encourages me to keep going, stand firm, and be strong. Our church members were so happy for me and my husband and the changes we were making. Then one day my son said, "Wow, Mom, you have muscles! You look great!" That was the ultimate compliment—to have my kids be supportive. Now we go on bike outings as a family and with our church family. What a blessing!

I have lost 39 pounds and kept it off for over a year. I used to crash by midday, but now I have energy throughout the entire day. This journey has been physical, mental, and spiritual. I love my new lifestyle!
Sincerely,
Roxanne

Be Positive

Plant seeds of good health and let them take root.

Be Fruitful

BREAKFAST: Something on the Go

Top ⅔ cup 1% cottage cheese with ½ cup cubed cantaloupe and 2 tablespoons chopped walnuts. Enjoy with 1 whole-wheat English muffin.

295 calories, 25 grams protein, 27 grams carbohydrate, 11 grams fat, 4 grams fiber

SNACK: Mixed Berry Dream Smoothie

In a blender, combine 1 serving Greenberry Shakeology (or 6 ounces of any low-sugar protein powder), 1 cup berries, ⅓ cup rice milk or almond milk, 1 cup water, and ice.

157 calories, 5 grams protein, 18 grams carbohydrate, 8 grams fat, 3 grams fiber

LUNCH: Dijon Tuna Salad

Combine 4 ounces drained water-packed white-meat tuna, ¼ cup chopped celery, and ¼ cup chopped green pepper with a mixture of 1 tablespoon Dijon mustard and 2 tablespoons low-fat mayonnaise. Scoop onto a large salad composed of 2 cups mixed greens, 1 cup red and green pepper strips, ⅓ sliced cucumber, and 5 cherry tomatoes. Serve with 3 pieces whole-wheat melba toast and either a fresh peach or ½ cup sliced peaches canned in juice, drained.

401 calories, 31 grams protein, 42 grams carbohydrate, 13 grams fat, 10 grams fiber

SNACK: Herbed Cheese and Turkey

Top 5 whole-wheat crackers (should total about 50 calories) with 1 tablespoon spreadable herb cheese (like Laughing Cow) and 1½ ounces deli turkey breast. Serve with 1 small sliced red pepper.

144 calories, 12 grams of protein, 15 grams carbohydrate, 5 grams fat, 3 grams fiber

DINNER: Jerk Chicken

Prepare rub by mixing together 1 tablespoon apple cider vinegar, ½ teaspoon ground allspice, ½ teaspoon ground cloves, ½ teaspoon thyme, and ¼ teaspoon each of salt and pepper. Coat 3 ounces of chicken breast meat with rub. Bake at 400°F until cooked through (approximately 25 minutes). Serve with a small baked sweet potato and a mixed green salad tossed with 2 teaspoons olive oil and 2 tablespoons fresh lime juice.

387 calories, 31 grams protein, 38 grams carbohydrate, 13 grams fat, 6 grams fiber

Be Joyful

SONG OF THE DAY: "Baby I'm a Star" by Prince

Be Fit

WARM-UP: 3–5 minutes

CARDIO AND STRENGTH TRAINING: Burn, Baby, Burn

STRETCH: 3–5 minutes

Burn, Baby, Burn Workout

Jump Rope

Exercise 1
Stand straight with a rope in your hands. Jump rope by hopping from one foot to the other. Perform for 1 minute. (This exercise can be done without the rope.)

Pull-Up

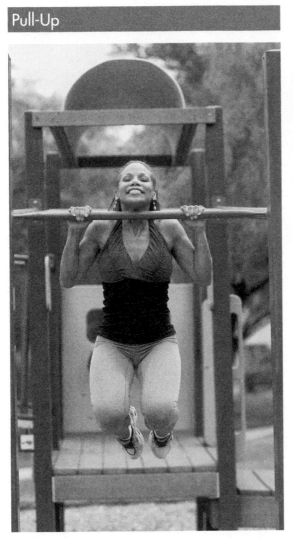

Lunge Jump

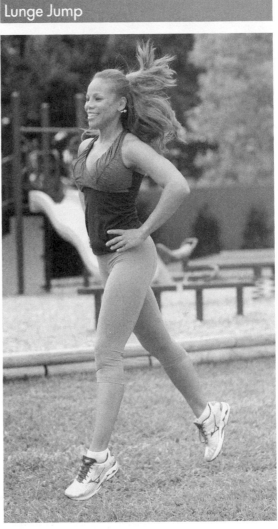

Exercise 2

Find some monkey bars, a sturdy tree branch, or a well-secured pull-up bar that is low enough that your hands can touch the bar. Jump up and grab the bar with your knees bent. Pull your chest above the bar, then lower yourself down and land with both feet on the ground. Repeat. Perform for 1 minute.

Exercise 3

Stand tall and step into a lunge position with your hands on your hips. Jump straight up and switch your feet, landing on the other side. Repeat. Perform for 1 minute.

Decline Push-Up

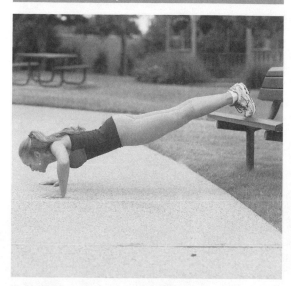

Exercise 4

Start in a push-up position with your feet on a chair or bench and your arms extended. Tighten your abs, bend your elbows, and lower your chest to the ground. Keep your body in a straight line. Push yourself back up to the starting position and repeat. Perform for 1 minute.

Squat Jump

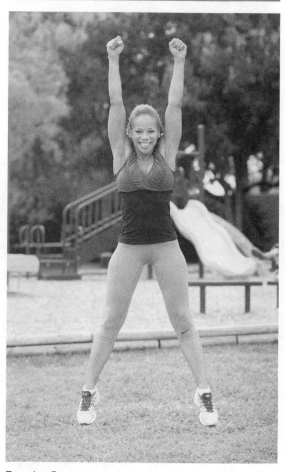

Exercise 5

Stand tall with your feet hip-width apart and lower yourself to a squat position. Jump straight up, with your arms extended straight up above your head. Land in a squat position and repeat. Perform for 1 minute.

Tricep Push-Up

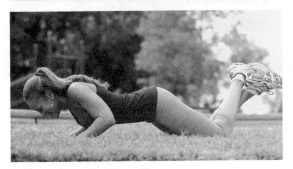

Exercise 6

Start on your hands and knees with your hands close together. Lower your chest to the ground, keeping your body in line and your elbows bent back. Push up by straightening your arms back to the starting position. Perform for 1 minute.

Optional: For a more demanding workout, perform this exercise with your legs straight.

Suicide Shuffle

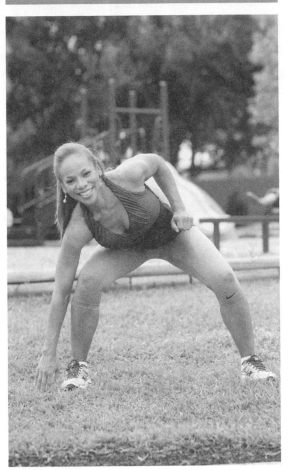

Exercise 7

Stand tall with your feet hip-width apart. Bend your legs, lowering yourself into a squat position and lifting onto the balls of your feet. Staying on the balls of your feet, shuffle to one side for three counts, then extend the hand on the same side to the ground on the fourth count. Shuffle to the other side and repeat. Perform for 1 minute.

Wood Chopper

Exercise 8

Stand with your feet shoulder-width apart, your hands clasped together, and your arms bent above shoulder level. Contract your abs and lower yourself into a squat position. Swing your arms diagonally across your body toward your right leg. Push through your heels and raise your body up while lifting your bent arms above your head and returning to the start position. Alternate sides and repeat for 1 minute.

Optional: For a more demanding workout, hold a medicine ball or weights in your hands.

REPEAT CIRCUIT 2–3 TIMES.

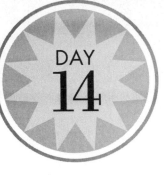
Be Faithful

Take delight in the Lord, and he will give
you the desires of your heart.
—PSALM 37:4

Be Grateful

BRENDA'S STORY

In January 2011, Brenda started working out and joined one of my fitness
clubs at her church. She had reached her heaviest weight, 278 pounds, and had
experienced her worst level of depression. She remembers her grandmother
rewarding her with food all the time as she was growing up. For years, Brenda
watched her mother go on and off diets as her weight went up and down.
Eventually, everyone in her family became diabetic and faced other serious health
concerns. Although Brenda continued to gain weight, she kept telling herself, "I'm
not going to be like my mother." But she had become just like her mother. When
it was time to attend her high school reunion, Brenda knew all her friends were
going, but she was ashamed and didn't want others to make fun of her or judge
her. She had just lost two cousins: one (age late forties) had died from a heart
attack and the other (age early fifties) from diabetic complications. Also fresh in
her memory was her last plane ride, when she had to ask for an extended seat
belt. She went into prayer and asked God to help her.

For many years, Brenda had self-medicated her depression with food. But her
depression was caused by her weight problem. Food was like a drug—the more
she had, the more she wanted. Her life revolved around food. Brenda prayed that
she would desire healthy foods and that gluttony would no longer be her sin.
Then she decided to try my plan. After six months of working out, tracking calorie
intake, being in the church program, and having a reliable support group, Brenda
lost 65 pounds and attended her high school reunion. She was happy about her
accomplishment, though she still felt under attack. Regardless, she continued
to charge ahead because she knew God was strengthening her so she could help

others. She and her husband became the co-leaders of a church program that consisted of working out, sharing tips, giving encouragement, and leading prayer. Every day she tells herself, "Don't tell God how big the problem is; tell the problem how big God is." She refuses to be defeated, and she is giving her all to get what she wants.

She has lost 108 pounds and is determined to reach her goal of losing 125 pounds overall. When her friend asked her what she would do if she was off by a few pounds on the day before her deadline, she replied, "I will participate in my own aerobic-thon all day long and reach my goal." Brenda has achieved and will continue to achieve her goals, and I'm grateful that she shares her story to help others be victors—and not victims—of their health.

Hallelujah!

Be Positive

Cherish your healthy relationships and be glad in the love and support you receive from loved ones.

Be Fruitful

BREAKFAST: Bacon and Cheese Scrambled Eggs

Spray a nonstick skillet with cooking spray and heat over medium heat. In a small bowl, beat 2 large eggs, 2 egg whites, 2 teaspoons vegetarian bacon bits, and 3 tablespoons fat-free milk. Pour the egg mixture into the skillet and scramble until almost set. Sprinkle ¼ cup low-fat cheddar cheese over the eggs, and continue to scramble until cooked to desired consistency. Transfer to a serving plate and enjoy with a ¼ cantaloupe wedge and 6 ounces apple juice.

390 calories, 31 grams protein, 38 grams carbohydrate, 14 grams fat, 2 grams fiber

SNACK: Salmon Salad on Crispbread

Wash ¼ medium tomato, peel ¼ cucumber, and slice both thinly. Drain 1 ounce salmon (canned in water) and combine with 1 teaspoon low-fat mayonnaise and ½ teaspoon Dijon mustard in a small bowl. Spread salmon salad onto 2 pieces rye low-sodium crispbread crackers; top with tomato and cucumber slices. Enjoy with 8 ounces water.

120 calories, 8 grams protein, 15 grams carbohydrate, 3.5 grams fat, 3 grams fiber

LUNCH: Mojito Shake

Combine 1 packet of Tropical Strawberry Shakeology mix (or 6 ounces of any low-sugar protein powder), 1 tablespoon fresh lime, 2 tablespoons chopped fresh mint leaves, 1 cup water, and ice to taste (add more ice for a thicker shake). Mix in blender until creamy.

> 166 calories, 15 grams protein, 22 grams carbohydrate,
> 1 gram fat, 3 grams fiber

SNACK: Pesto-Artichoke Chicken Wrap

Shred 2 tablespoons cooked chicken. In a small bowl, mix together shredded chicken, 2½ teaspoons coarsely chopped artichoke hearts (fresh, cooked, or canned), and ½ teaspoon fresh chopped scallions. Set aside.

Spread ½ teaspoon pesto sauce on a 6-inch low-carb tortilla. Arrange chicken mix and 1 pimento strip on top. Roll up tortilla; heat if desired. Have an 8-ounce glass of water.

> 120 calories, 9 grams protein, 13g carbohydrate,
> 3.5 grams fat, 8 grams fiber

DINNER: Broiled Mustard Steak

Spray a broiler pan rack with nonstick cooking spray. Preheat broiler. Trim any fat from 7 ounces beef tenderloin. Brush steak with 2 teaspoons extra-virgin olive oil. Season steak with ⅛ teaspoon salt and ¼ teaspoon black pepper. Mix together 1 tablespoon chopped green onion, 1 teaspoon Dijon mustard, and 1 teaspoon chopped garlic. Place the steak on the broiler pan rack, and broil 5 to 6 inches from heat for 4 to 5 minutes. Spread the top of the steak with half the mustard-onion mixture and broil for another 2 minutes. Turn the steak over and broil for another 4 to 5 minutes. Spread the top of the steak with the remaining mustard-onion mixture and broil for another 2 minutes, or to desired doneness. Let rest for 5 minutes before slicing and serving.

Spinach Salad

Halve 4 cherry tomatoes and toss with 1¼ cups fresh, chopped spinach and ¼ cup sliced mushrooms. Drizzle with 1½ teaspoons reduced-fat ranch dressing and 1 tablespoon balsamic vinegar.

Garlic Mashed Potatoes

Boil ⅞ cup diced potatoes until tender. Mash with 2 tablespoons fat-free, low-sodium chicken broth, 1 teaspoon trans-fat-free, canola-based margarine, and 1 teaspoon chopped garlic. Season with salt and pepper to taste.

Dessert: Enjoy 1 SnackWell's fat-free devil's food cookie cake and a tangerine

590 calories, 46 grams protein, 56 grams carbohydrate, 22 grams fat, 7 grams fiber

Be Joyful

SONG OF THE DAY: "I Feel Good" by James Brown

Be Fit

Weekly Fitness Diary

_____

_____

_____

_____

_____

_____

_____

_____

_____

_____

_____

_____

_____

_____

_____

Be Faithful

*Now to him that is able to do exceeding
abundantly above all that we ask or think,
according to the power that works in us.*
—EPHESIANS 3:20

Be Grateful

DION'S STORY

When I met Donna, I told her I was lacking in all areas of my life and needed
a full tune-up. My girlfriend, Doneice, and I signed up for Donna's program
because we wanted more than just a workout; we needed our bodies and souls
to be fed. Every day, five days a week, we showed up for class. The workout
was for us an extension of church, because we were able to worship while we
exercised. This was the most quality time we spent together because I worked a
night shift and she worked a day shift. At the time we joined the program our
relationship was shaky and we were in search of answers. I felt we were not as
one. We were always separated; even in church she worked with toddlers during
service. At home, we didn't eat or pray together. We were lost.

Every day our souls were being fed, yet we were thirsty for more. Yes, we were
depleted, but we strengthened our faith in God and in each other. The bonus
was losing the weight. I lost 80 pounds and Doneice lost 26 pounds. We were so
inspired by Donna, who would show up so peppy at 6:00 A.M., ready to pray,
work out, and share the word! If it wasn't for her program, I don't think Doneice
and I would have made it. We are now happily married, and I thank Donna for
attending our wedding. We now have a baby girl, Brooklyn.

I'm currently touring with a comedy show and pursuing an acting career.
My lifestyle has completely changed. I now realize that you have to know God to
know who you are and what his purpose and plan is for your life.

Dion

Be Positive

Remember you are fearfully and wonderfully made and all things are possible!

Be Fruitful

BREAKFAST: Cereal with Raspberries and Walnuts

Pour ¾ cup whole-grain cereal into a bowl and add 1 cup (8 ounces) fat-free milk, 1½ tablespoons chopped walnuts, and ⅓ cup raspberries. Enjoy with 1 strip of low-fat string cheese on the side. Serve with a cup of coffee or tea, lightened with ½ cup (4 ounces) milk.

> 420 calories, 28 grams protein, 50 grams carbohydrate, 15 grams fat, 8 grams fiber

SNACK: Hard-Boiled Egg

Enjoy a large hard-boiled egg and ½ small banana for this quick snack.

> 120 calories, 7 grams protein, 12 grams carbohydrate, 5 grams fat, 1 gram fiber

LUNCH: Shakeology Cranberry Chiller

Combine one packet of Greenberry Shakeology mix (or 6 ounces of any low-sugar protein powder), ½ cup unsweetened cranberry juice, 1 cup water, and ice to taste (add more ice for a thicker shake). Mix in blender until creamy.

> 198 calories, 15 grams protein, 34 grams carbohydrate, 0.5 grams fat, 3 grams fiber

SNACK: Beef Jerky

Enjoy ¾ ounce California-style, teriyaki-flavored beef jerky, 2 whole-wheat crackers, and 8 ounces water for this simple snack.

> 130 calories, 11 grams protein, 15 grams carbohydrate, 3.5 grams fat, 2 grams fiber

DINNER: Basil Chicken

Preheat oven to 425°F. Spray a shallow baking dish with nonstick cooking spray. In a food processor or blender, combine 2 tablespoons fresh chopped basil leaves, 1 ounce fat-free, low-sodium chicken broth, 1½ teaspoons chopped garlic, 2 teaspoons extra-virgin olive oil, ⅛ teaspoon ground thyme, ⅛ teaspoon black pepper, and ⅛ teaspoon salt. Process until pureed. Place 6½ ounces boneless, skinless chicken breast in the baking dish and rub both sides with the basil mixture. Bake for 20 to 25 minutes, or until chicken is no longer pink inside.

Three Bean Salad

Toss ¼ cup cooked green beans, ¼ cup cooked yellow beans, and 2 tablespoons canned, reduced-sodium kidney beans with 2 tablespoons cider vinegar and ⅛ teaspoon fresh cracked black pepper. Refrigerate until ready to serve.

Quick and Easy Couscous

Prepare couscous per package directions. Portion out ⅔ cup. Drizzle with ¾ teaspoon extra-virgin olive oil and ½ teaspoon fresh chopped parsley.

Dessert: Blueberries

Top 1 cup blueberries with 2 tablespoons fat-free whipped topping and enjoy for dessert.

> 590 calories, 46 grams protein, 60 grams carbohydrate,
> 3 grams fat, 10 grams fiber

Be Joyful

SONG OF THE DAY: "I Smile" by Kirk Franklin

Be Fit

WARM-UP: 3–5 minutes

CARDIO: 30–60 minutes

STRENGTH TRAINING AND STRETCHING: Wit 2 Fit Yoga

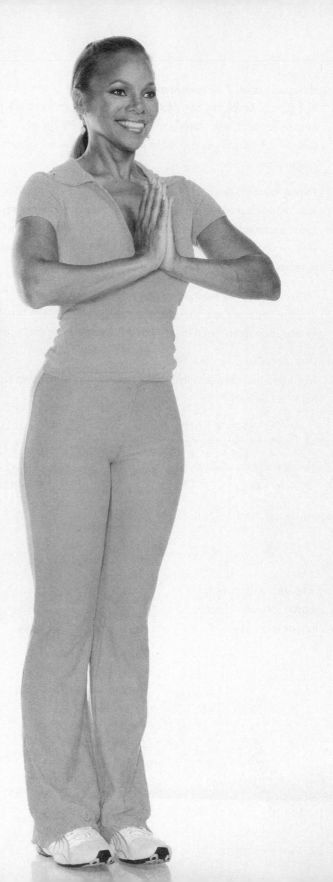

Wit 2 Fit Yoga Workout

Mountain Pose

Exercise 1

Stand tall with your feet together and your arms by your sides. Bring your hands to your heart. Inhale and exhale through your nose 5 times.

Standing Forward Bend

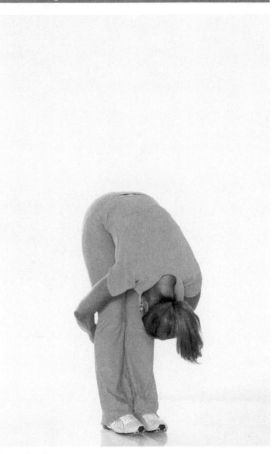

Modified Warrior 1

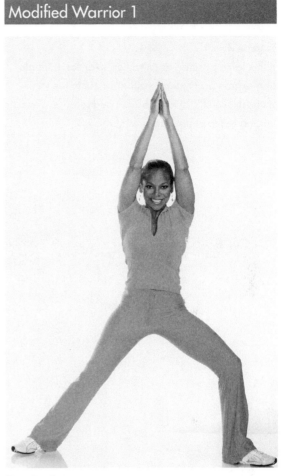

Exercise 2

Stand tall with your feet together and your arms at your sides. Inhale, reaching your hands to the ceiling. Then exhale while bending at the waist, allowing your upper body to relax. (*Optional:* hold your calves.) Hold for 5 breaths.

Exercise 3

Stand tall with your feet together and your hands at your sides. Inhale and lift your left leg into a lunge position with your left foot turned out and your left knee bent. Keep your hips squared to the front and extend your arms above your head with your palms together. Hold for 1 breath. Repeat, lunging to the right.

Modified Warrior 2

Exercise 4

In the same position as Modified Warrior 1, inhale, then exhale and extend your arms out to the sides at chest level. Hold for 1 breath and release. Repeat, lunging to the other side.

Extended Triangle

Exercise 5

Take the same starting position as before—a lunge. Inhale as you straighten your front leg, then exhale as you extend one arm alongside your leg and extend the other arm toward the ceiling while bending your front knee. Hold for 1 breath and release. Switch sides and repeat.

Lifted Triangle

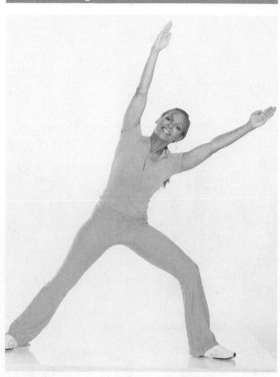

Chair Pose

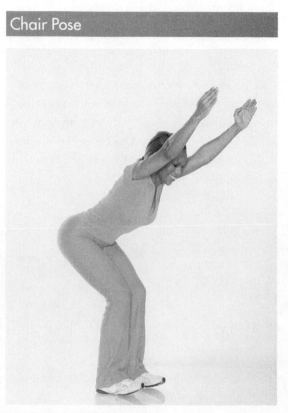

Exercise 6

Take the same starting position as before—a lunge. Reach your arms above your head diagonally. Hold for 1 breath and release. Switch sides and repeat.

Exercise 7

Stand with your feet together. Inhale and lower your tailbone toward the floor while you extend your arms above your head, keeping your knees over your toes. Keep your abs tight and back straight, and tuck in your tailbone, like you are sitting down in a chair. Hold for 5–10 breaths.

Standing Chest Lift

Exercise 8

Exhale and place your hands on your hips. Lift your chest toward the ceiling as you push your elbows back and together. Press your hips forward and arch your back. Hold for 5–10 breaths.

REPEAT CIRCUIT 1–2 TIMES.

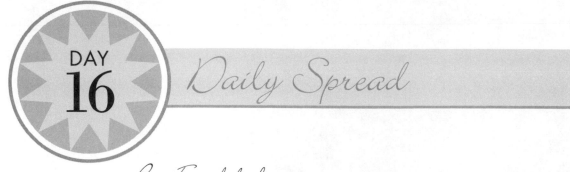

Be Faithful

*I press on toward the goal to win the prize for which
God has called me heavenward in Christ Jesus.*
—PHILIPPIANS 3:14

Be Grateful

CAROL'S STORY

*I met Carol through her daughter, Wanda, who works with me in our quest to
deliver a message of hope and health around the world. As the mother of three
grown daughters, Carol had much motivation and encouragement to get fit.
Wanda and her two sisters, Cheri and Wendi, didn't want to see their mother
encountering more health problems and she did not want to continue being
stressed out and depressed about her weight, so they all decided to start my
program. In addition, Carol's brother told her he would buy her a new wardrobe
if she achieved her goal weight. Having failed at other weight-loss programs and
gimmicky solutions, Carol was hesitant to try again, but she did it anyway. She
was sick and tired of feeling sick and tired.*

*Together with her daughters, Carol started eating healthy and working out
with my exercise DVDs. In fact, Carol's passion to get fit was inspired by her
daughter Wendi. Carol never gave up, and neither did Wendi. Now, Wendi is 40
pounds lighter! They also incorporated using resistance bands and walking on
a treadmill into their workouts. After only six months, Carol had lost 30 pounds
but gained so much. Her blood pressure had gone down and she had increased
mobility. Carol also now has a new attitude. Her goal? She wants to lose another
20 pounds by the end of the year and fit comfortably into a size 12. And that's not
all! She says with a smile, "Now that I'm losing all of this weight, I might want to
find a man!"*

Though this journey hasn't always been an easy one, Carol admits it has been well worth the effort. Now when she travels, she no longer has to get a skycap to take her to and from her gate. She is able to walk through the airport with her head held high and without getting winded. She finds she can exercise longer, and she can perform daily tasks such as cleaning, cooking, and yard work much more easily than before. And she's really looking forward to shopping for new clothes in her smaller size.

Carol is an inspiration to all who encounter her. She says, "It's never too late to get fit!"

Be Positive

Keep the goal in sight and keep pressing on. Remember, every step you take brings you closer to your dreams!

Be Fruitful

BREAKFAST: Shakeology Mocha Chiller

Blend 1 packet of Chocolate Shakeology mix (or 6 ounces of any low-sugar protein powder), 1 cup cold coffee, and ice to taste (add more ice for a thicker shake). Mix in blender until creamy.

142 calories, 17 grams protein, 17 grams carbohydrate, 1 gram fat, 3 grams fiber

SNACK: Soy Nuts and Raisins

Enjoy a mixture of 1½ tablespoons unsalted, dry-roasted soy bean nuts and 2 teaspoons raisins.

100 calories, 6 grams protein, 11 grams carbohydrate, 4 grams fat, 3 grams fiber

LUNCH: Roast Beef on Rye

Spread 1 tablespoon low-fat mayonnaise onto 1 slice rye bread. Arrange 3½ ounces lean, deli-style roast beef, ½ medium sliced tomato, and 1 lettuce leaf on bread. Serve open-faced sandwich with a small glass (4 ounces) of fat-free milk.

290 calories, 25 grams protein, 29 grams carbohydrate, 8 grams fat, 3 grams fiber

SNACK: Turkey Lettuce Wrap

Wash 1 lettuce leaf and pat dry with a paper towel; set aside. Wash
¼ medium tomato and either chop finely or slice thinly. Spread 1 teaspoon
low-fat mayonnaise evenly onto one side of a slice of oven-roasted fat-free
low-sodium turkey breast. On top, place lettuce leaf, tomato, and another
2 ounces turkey, and roll up from one end into a full roll-up. Secure roll with a
toothpick, if desired. Enjoy with 6 baby carrots.

90 calories, 11 grams protein, 7 grams carbohydrate, 2 grams fat, 2 grams fiber

DINNER: Scrumptious Salmon Cakes

Use 5½ ounces salmon, either canned in water and drained, or
salmon in a pouch, or leftover cooked salmon. Wash and finely chop
1 tablespoon green onion and 1½ tablespoons red bell pepper.
In a medium bowl, gently flake the salmon. Stir in red bell pepper,
green onion, ½ tablespoon mayonnaise, 1 tablespoon fat-free sour
cream, 1 tablespoon lemon juice, and ⅛ teaspoon black pepper. Add
1 tablespoon cornflake crumbs and 2 tablespoons liquid egg substitute
to salmon mixture, mixing thoroughly to combine. Divide and form
mixture into 2 small balls, then flatten into cakes approximately ¼ inch
thick. Sauté cakes over medium-high heat in a skillet coated with nonstick
cooking spray until golden brown on both sides.

For lemon-herb sauce, mix together 1 tablespoon sour cream,
1 tablespoon lemon juice, and ⅛ teaspoon ground thyme. Drizzle
over salmon cakes.

Tuscan Penne Pasta

Prepare ⅔ cup plain penne pasta per package directions. Drain and
rinse. Cut 1 tablespoon sun-dried tomatoes (not in oil) into strips. Toss
⅔ cup cooked pasta with ½ teaspoon extra-virgin olive oil, ⅛ teaspoon
black pepper, 2 teaspoons fresh, chopped basil, tomatoes, and ¼ ounce
reduced-fat (50% less fat) goat cheese (¼ ounce equals 1 tablespoon).

Dessert: Raspberries

Enjoy a large bowl of raspberries (1½ cups) for dessert.

> 620 calories, 44 grams protein, 65 grams carbohydrate,
> 21 grams fat, 14 grams fiber

Be Joyful

SONG OF THE DAY: "Long Train Running" by the Doobie Brothers

Be Fit

WARM-UP: 3–4 minutes

CARDIO: Rocking Walking

STRENGTH TRAINING: 10–20 minutes

STRETCH: 3–5 minutes

Rocking Walking Workout

Alternating Knee Hop

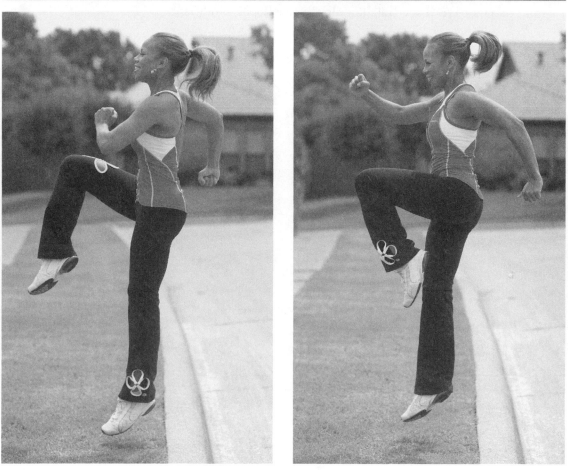

Position A

Position B

Walk for 4 minutes. Face a curb while marching in place. Step up and push off with one foot while lifting the opposite knee and keeping your hands bent at your sides (Position A). Step down off the curb with the foot of the bent knee, then step up and push off with the opposite foot (Position B). Step down to the starting position. Alternate sides and perform for 1 minute.

Sidewalk Hop

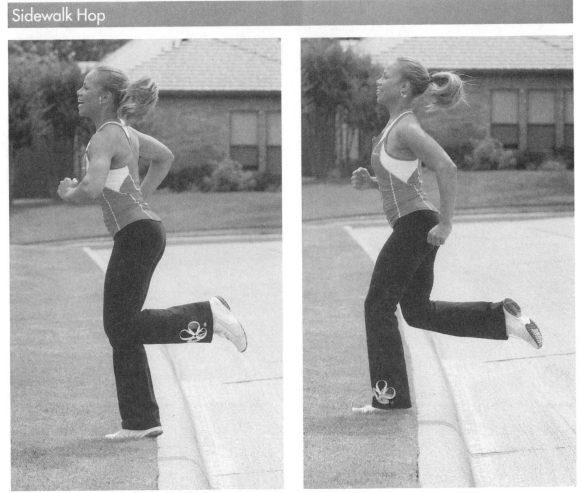

Position A   **Position B**

Walk for 4 minutes, then face the curb. Hop on the right foot onto the sidewalk (Position A), then hop with the left foot onto the sidewalk (Position B). Step down with the right foot, then with the left foot. Perform for 1 minute.

Curbside Jump

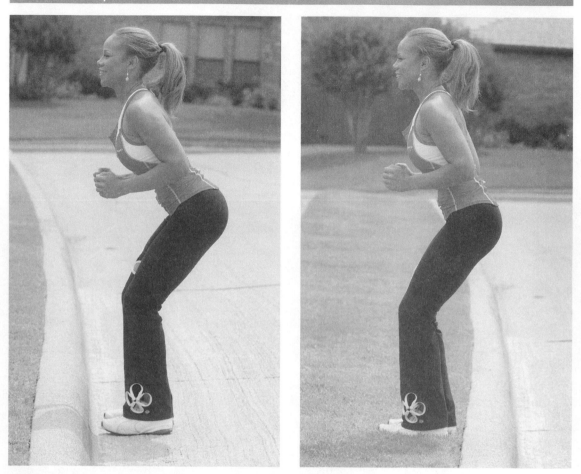

Position A

Position B

Walk for 4 minutes, then face the curb (Position A). Jump up with both feet (Position B), then step down with one foot, then the other. Perform for 1 minute.

Leg Lift

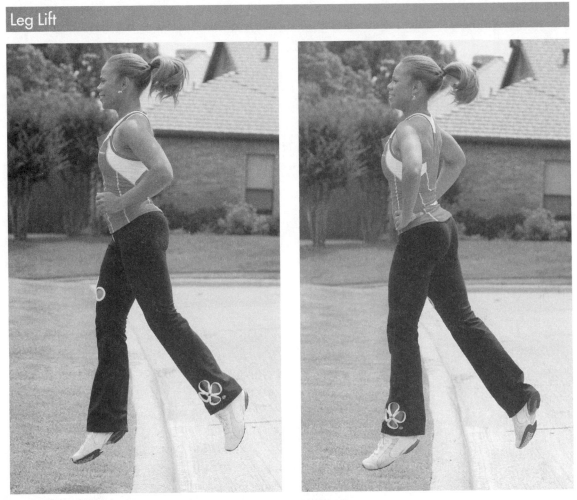

Position A   **Position B**

Walk for 4 minutes, then face the curb. Step and jump with your right foot onto the curb, lifting your left leg back and keeping your arms bent at your sides (Position A). Then step back down off the curb. Switch legs, then step and jump onto the curb with your left foot, lifting your right leg back and keeping your arms bent at your sides (Position B). Alternate sides. Perform for 1 minute.

THE FULL CYCLE TAKES 20 MINUTES; DO 2–3 TIMES.

Workouts may be performed indoors with a step or an exercise step stool.

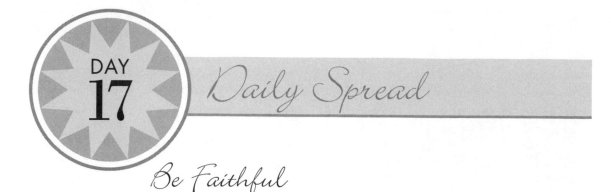

Be Faithful

*Now faith is the substance of things hoped for,
the evidence of things not seen.*

—HEBREWS 11:1

Be Grateful

WALTER'S STORY

Walter was diagnosed with multiple sclerosis (MS) at age thirty-nine. MS is an inflammatory disease that affects the ability of the nerve cells in the brain and the spinal cord to communicate effectively. When Walter got the diagnosis, he broke down in tears, asking in his anger, "Why me?" He was at the top of his career as one of lead singers for the legendary R&B group the O'Jays. Walter's singing made women scream and throw their panties onto the stage.

Because of the disease, Walter's feet and toes became numb, his motor skills dwindled, his balance became unstable, he gained weight, and his life expectancy was at best twenty years. Once a week for thirteen years he got a shot in the hip that gave him flu-like symptoms, extreme headaches, and nausea to the point of not being able to perform, but God made a way.

Faced with a disease that could end his career, his dreams, even his life, he told himself, "I'm fighting. I'm not going down without a fight." He decided not to tell anyone but family and group members about the MS, because he didn't want people to feel sorry for him. He has been exercising and eating healthier for many years, and in the past year he hasn't taken any medication for MS. He admits that at times he was afraid, but he never lost sight of his faith. What he once saw as a curse has actually been a blessing in disguise.

Although he didn't want to be handicapped by the disease, Walter now enjoys having a good handicap. He has become an avid golfer and any time he can go out and play, he is grateful for that moment.

Be Positive

Let go of past hurts and barriers. Move on and
be free. It's time to forgive and live.

Be Fruitful

BREAKFAST: French Toast and Sausage

Mix ¼ cup liquid egg substitute and ¼ teaspoon ground cinnamon in a bowl;
soak 2 pieces whole-wheat bread until liquid is absorbed. Heat a nonstick
skillet lightly coated with cooking spray over medium-high heat. Place egg-
soaked bread on hot skillet; cook both sides until lightly browned. Top with
¼ cup blueberries and 2 teaspoons powdered sugar. Prepare 2 pieces turkey
breakfast sausage according to package instructions, and serve on the side.
Enjoy a small (4 ounces) glass of fat-free milk with breakfast.

> 400 calories, 32 grams protein, 40 grams carbohydrate,
> 13 grams fat, 5 grams fiber

SNACK: Chicken Salad

Shred 2½ tablespoons cooked chicken breast. Mix chicken with 1 teaspoon
low-fat mayonnaise and ⅛ teaspoon dried dill weed. Serve with (or on)
1 piece thin-sliced whole-wheat bread. Enjoy with an 8-ounce glass of water.

> 120 calories, 9 grams protein, 11 grams carbohydrate,
> 3.5 grams fat, 2 grams fiber

LUNCH: Watermelon Wave Shake

Blend 1 packet of Tropical Strawberry Shakeology mix (or 6 ounces of any
low-sugar protein powder), ½ cup chopped watermelon, 1 cup water, and
ice to taste (add more ice for a thicker shake). Mix in blender until creamy.

> 183 calories, 15.5 grams protein, 26 grams carbohydrate,
> 1 gram fat, 3 grams fiber

SNACK: Cottage Cheese and Strawberries

Top ⅓ cup 1% cottage cheese with 6 whole fresh strawberries and 1½
teaspoons chopped pecans.

Enjoy with an 8-ounce glass of water.

> 110 calories, 9 grams protein, 13 grams carbohydrate,
> 35 grams fat, 2 grams fiber

DINNER: Sweet Pepper Pork

Place 6 ounces boneless pork sirloin chops between two pieces of plastic wrap. Using a wooden mallet, pound to ⅛-inch thickness. Remove plastic wrap. Heat 1½ teaspoons extra-virgin olive oil over medium-high heat and cook the pork slice for 2 to 4 minutes, or until meat is browned and juices run clear, turning over once. Remove from skillet and keep warm. Cut ¼ yellow onion and ½ medium green bell pepper into thin strips and slice 4 fresh mushrooms. Add onion, bell pepper, mushrooms, ½ teaspoon chopped garlic, and ¼ teaspoon cumin to skillet and cook approximately 4 minutes or until vegetables are crisp-tender. Serve vegetable mixture with pork slice.

Broccoli

Steam 4 broccoli spears on stove or in microwave until crisp-tender. Top with ½ teaspoon low-fat melted buttery spread.

Brown Rice

Prepare ½ cup brown rice per package directions. Drizzle with ¾ teaspoon sesame oil and top with 1 teaspoon chopped green onions.

Dessert: Quick Blueberry Crisp

Melt ¼ teaspoon unsalted butter. Crush 1 graham cracker (2½-inch square); combine crumbs with butter and ½ teaspoon packed brown sugar. Set aside. Place ⅓ cup blueberries in a small microwave-safe bowl. Top with crumb mixture. Microwave on high for 30 seconds or until heated and bubbly. Top with 1 teaspoon fat-free whipped topping.

620 calories, 45 grams protein, 60 grams carbohydrate, 23 grams fat, 8 grams fiber

Be Joyful

SONG OF THE DAY: "Respect" by Aretha Franklin

Be Fit

WARM-UP: 3–5 minutes
CARDIO: 30–60 minutes
STRENGTH TRAINING: Lovely Legs
STRETCH: 3–5 minutes

Lovely Legs Workout

Dead Leg Lift

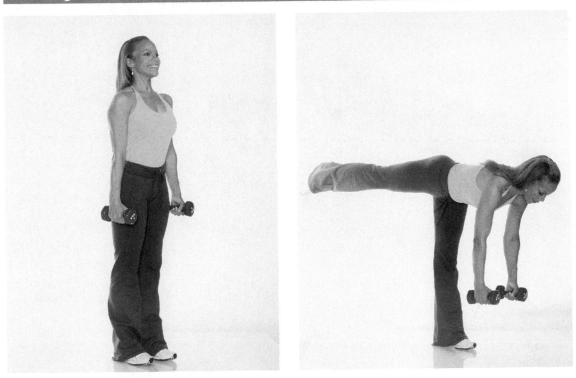

Position A

Position B

Stand tall with your feet slightly apart, holding weights in your hands with your arms at your sides (Position A). Contract your abs, bending forward at the waist until you are parallel to the floor while keeping your back straight. Let your arms hang down from your shoulders and lift one leg behind you (Position B). Then return to the starting position. Perform 12–15 reps, then switch to the other leg.

Plank Lunge and Row

Start in a full-body push-up position while holding weights in your hands. Bring your left knee up toward your chest (Position A), then extend it back to the starting position. Lift your right elbow with the weight in your hand toward the ceiling (Position B), then lower it back to the starting position. Perform 12–15 reps, then repeat on the other side.

Position A

Position B

Single-Leg Squat with Bicep Curl

Stand tall with your feet slightly apart, your right leg bent with the ball of your foot resting on the floor, and weights in your hands. Squat (right foot should lift off the floor), lifting the weight in your left hand up to the shoulder (Position A). Stand up straight, lifting your right leg to a knee lift, lowering your left hand to your side, and curling your right hand to the shoulder (Position B). Lower back into a squat position and repeat. Perform 12–15 reps, then repeat on the other side.

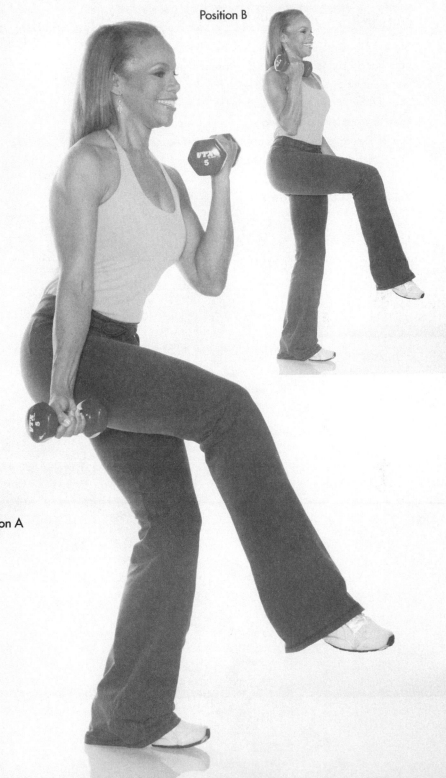

Position B

Position A

Side Lunge with Shoulder Press and Knee Lift

Stand tall with your feet slightly apart and weights in your hands. Lunge to the left side, raising the weights up with your elbows bent at chest level (Position A). Push off your left foot to return to a standing position, lifting your knee to waist level and lifting your arms to the sky (Position B). Return to the starting position and repeat on the opposite side. Perform 12–15 reps.

REPEAT CIRCUIT 1–3 TIMES.

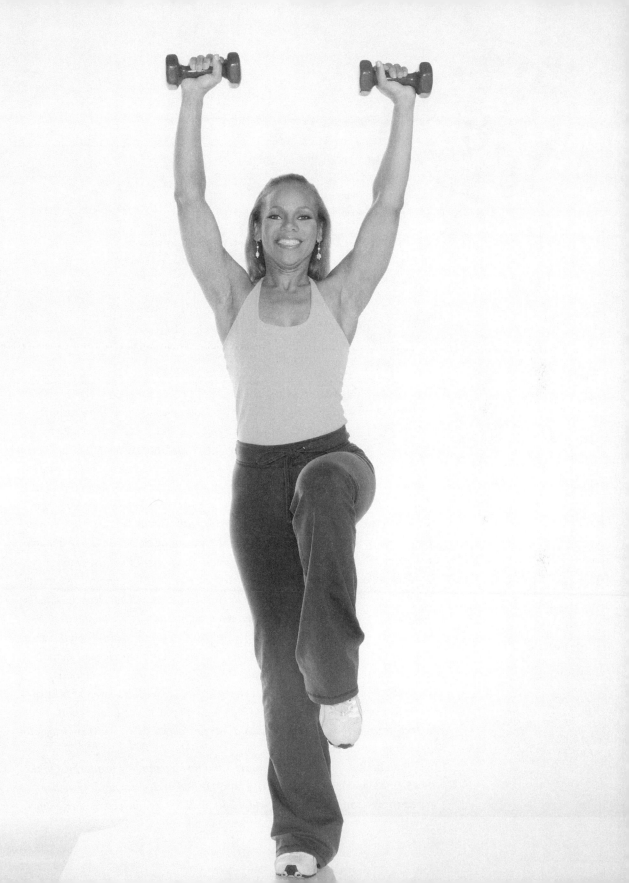

Be Faithful

*I will praise you; for I am fearfully and wonderfully made:
marvelous are your works; and that my soul knows right well.*
—PSALM 139:14

Be Grateful

TEDY'S STORY

*Last March, I climbed Mount Kilimanjaro. Soon thereafter, a fellow council
member on the President's Council for Fitness, Sports, and Nutrition, Tedy
Bruschi, climbed the mountain along with former Titans coach Jeff Fisher, former
Eagles tight end Chad Lewis, and four injured marines who climbed to raise
awareness of the Wounded Warrior Project. I had experienced firsthand what
it took to climb that mountain, and I was so inspired to hear the story of these
soldiers—two single-leg amputees, a marine with posttraumatic stress disorder,
and a soldier with only one eye—trekking and scaling the mountain. Although
two of the marines had to turn back, the journey changed their lives forever.*

*They called themselves Team Hard Target, and their mission was to conquer
the tallest freestanding mountain in the world. Guides and porters helped them
successfully navigate the wilderness. On a mountain, there are moments of
solitude where you hear only your breathing and nature's music. Then there was
their group experience. Tedy relates that they shared life experiences, football
stories, and counseling sessions, and their souls became one. Through this
incredible bonding experience you learn a lot about yourself as well as your co-
mountaineers. No matter how grueling the climb got, they told one another not
to look down the side of that mountain—the exact words my Kilimanjaro group
held on to during our climb.*

*On summit day, Tedy was exhausted and had a pounding headache. On the
way to the summit it was still pitch-black. He had been carrying Soldier Ben's
prosthetic leg and his own fifty-pound backpack. He had helped Soldier Nancy,*

who had lost her right eye in the Iraq War and had limited vision and depth
perception, change her socks to prevent frostbitten toes. And all he could focus on
was putting one foot in front of the other—left, right, left. As he continued his
ascent, a huge ray of hope appeared in the sky: sunrise! The sunrise became more
amazing with each step. It was the most beautiful and magical sight that he had
ever seen in his life.

As they finished the final fifty yards together, they rejoiced and congratulated
each other for this achievement of a lifetime. It gives hope and strength to believe
in the impossible and do the unthinkable.

Be Positive

Be a grateful and humble person and give thanks for the
little things that we sometimes take for granted.

Be Fruitful

BREAKFAST: Irish Omelet

Cook a medium potato (2½ to 3 inches) in salted water until tender. Peel and
mash ¾ of the cooked potato with ½ teaspoon unsalted butter in a medium-
size bowl. Set aside. Separate 2 jumbo eggs. Beat the yolks until smooth. Add
the yolks to the mashed potato and mix well. Add ½ teaspoon lemon juice,
1½ teaspoons fresh chives, 1½ teaspoons fresh chopped scallions, ⅛ teaspoon
salt, and ¼ teaspoon black pepper. Beat egg whites until stiff. Fold into the
potato mixture. Spray an ovenproof skillet with nonstick cooking spray and
cook the potato mixture over medium-low heat.

Cook the omelet for about 3 minutes, or until bottom is set. Finish the
omelet under the broiler, cooking until top is set, color is golden brown, and
the omelet "puffs." Allow to cool for a minute or two, then flip onto a serving
plate and serve with 1½ tablespoons fat-free sour cream. Enjoy breakfast with
an 8-ounce glass of fat-free milk.

> 410 calories, 28 grams protein, 44 grams carbohydrate,
> 12 grams fat, 3 grams fiber

SNACK: Crunchy Ham, Cheese, and Veggie Stacks

Spread 1 teaspoon low-fat mayonnaise on a low-sodium rye crispbread
cracker. Arrange ⅓ sliced carrot and ¼ sliced cucumber on crispbread; top
with ½ ounce lean, reduced-sodium ham and 1 slice low-fat Swiss cheese.

Sprinkle with sodium-free spices and herbs of choice, such as freshly ground black pepper. Enjoy with a calorie-free beverage.

120 calories, 9 grams protein, 12 grams carbohydrate,
3.5 grams fat, 3 grams fiber

LUNCH: Strawberry Cheesecake Shake

Combine 1 packet of Greenberry Shakeology mix (or 6 ounces of any low-sugar protein powder), 1 ounce light cream cheese, 1 cup strawberries, ½ cup almond milk, ½ cup water, and ice to taste (add more ice for a thicker shake). Mix in blender until creamy.

349 calories, 20 grams protein, 43.5 grams carbohydrate,
5.5 grams fat, 3 grams fiber

SNACK: Edamame

Crunch on ½ cup steamed or boiled edamame for this easy snack. Serve with an 8-ounce glass of water.

100 calories, 8 grams protein, 9 grams carbohydrate,
3 grams fat, 4 grams fiber

DINNER: Glazed Chicken

Preheat oven to 375°F. Place 6½ ounces boneless, skinless chicken breast in a shallow baking dish coated with 1¼ teaspoons extra-virgin olive oil. For glaze, in a small bowl whisk with a fork 2 teaspoons packed brown sugar, 2 tablespoons orange juice, 1 teaspoon mustard (any flavor), 1 teaspoon fresh, chopped parsley, and a dash (⅛ teaspoon) of black pepper. Brush the glaze over the chicken. Bake chicken for 20 to 30 minutes, or until chicken is no longer pink.

Grilled Eggplant

Heat grill. Slice ¼ eggplant about ½ inch thick. Brush both sides of eggplant slices with ½ teaspoon extra-virgin olive oil. Season with salt and pepper. Place eggplant slices on the hot grill. Grill about 15 to 20 minutes, turning once.

Biscuit

Prepare two 2¼-inch low-fat buttermilk biscuits per package directions; top with ¾ teaspoon canola-based trans-fat-free margarine.

Dessert: Raspberries

Enjoy a large bowl (1½ cups) of raspberries for dessert.

600 calories, 44 grams protein, 67 grams carbohydrate,
170 grams fat, 18 grams fiber

Be Joyful

SONG OF THE DAY: "The Sky Is the Limit" by Virtue

Be Fit

WARM-UP: 3–5 minutes

CARDIO: 30–60 minutes

STRENGTH TRAINING: Wobble, Wobble Before You Gobble, Gobble

STRETCH: 3–5 minutes

Wobble, Wobble Before You Gobble, Gobble Workout

Squat Swing and Leg Lift

Stand with your feet slightly more than shoulder-width apart. Hold a weight in your hands and bend forward at the waist (Position A). Stand up straight and lift one leg to the side while you raise your arms above your head (Position B). Lower your leg and arms and return to the forward bend. Perform 15 reps, then repeat on the other side.

Position A

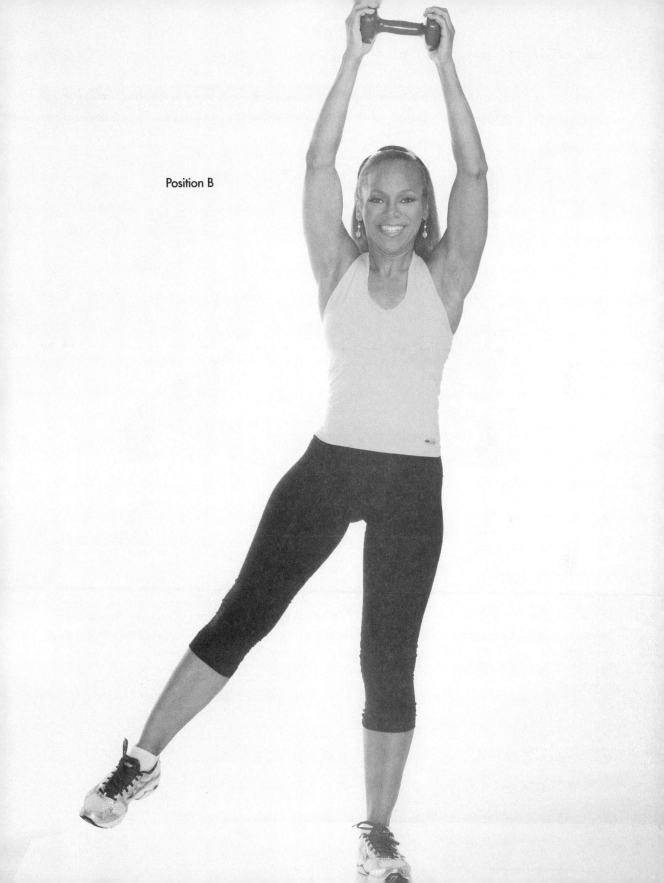

Position B

Lunge and Torso Twist

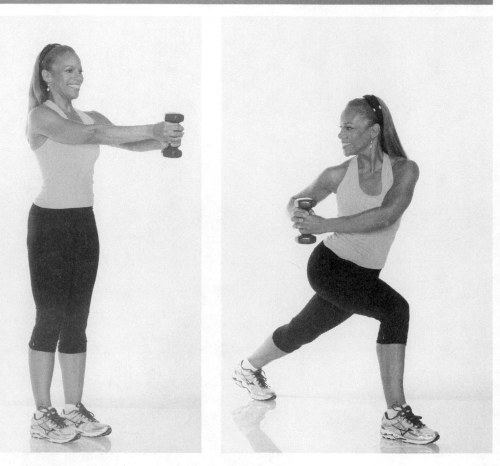

Position A

Position B

Stand with your feet slightly apart, holding a weight in your hands with your arms extended in front at chest level (Position A). Lunge back with your left leg, contract your abs, and rotate your torso to face the right (Position B). Rotate back to the center and return to the starting position. Perform 15 reps, then switch sides.

Hip Extension and Rear Deltoid

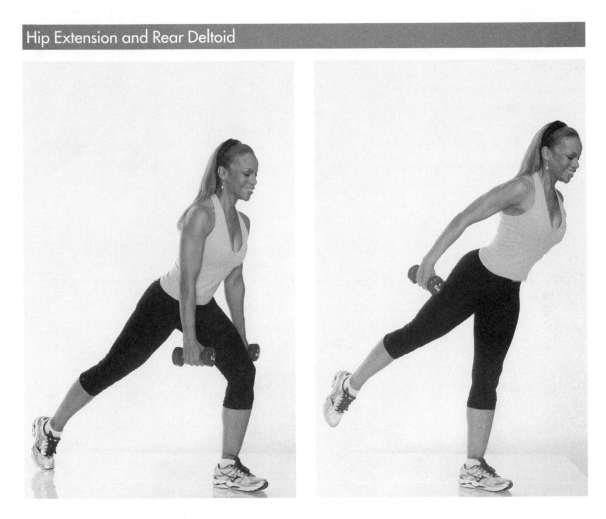

Position A

Position B

Start tall with your feet slightly apart. Lean slightly forward and lunge with your left leg forward, allowing your arms to hang down (Position A). Lift up your right leg and simultaneously extend your arms straight back (Position B). Return your right foot to the floor and return your arms to the front. Return to the starting position. Repeat on the opposite side. Perform 15 reps.

Plié, Calf Raise, and Bicep Curl

Stand tall with your feet slightly more than hip-width apart, your toes pointed outward, weights in your hands, and your arms hanging by your sides (Position A). Roll up onto the balls of your feet, bend your knees, and raise your arms to shoulder height (Position B). Return to the starting position. Perform 15 reps.

REPEAT CIRCUIT 1–3 TIMES.

Position B

Position A

Be Faithful

*You are of God, little children, and have
overcome them: because greater is he that is in
you, than he that is in the world.*

—1 JOHN 4:4

Be Grateful

AVIS'S STORY

On May 5, 2010, Avis's husband, James, felt a lump on her breast. The next day she visited her doctor to have a mammogram. She had had a mammogram a few months before and the results had been negative. This time, however, she was diagnosed with breast cancer. She sat motionless and said to herself, "I have cancer." She told her husband, who fell to his knees and started crying, but not one tear fell from her eyes. Four days later, no longer in shock, Avis took a leave of absence from work and set things in order.

When Avis went through chemotherapy, she had moments when she wanted to give up. The pain was unbearable, and she felt weak. It was horrific. But Avis, the fighter who had been taught by her father to never give up, asked God to walk with her through this ordeal because she wanted to live for her kids. She remembers that one morning, when she was holding on to a strand of hope, she started praying, as was customary for her. This time, she felt a gush of air through her mouth, then throughout her entire body. She knew then that she would be okay. She said, "Thank you, Jesus." After months of chemotherapy and radiation, she has now been cancer-free for six months.

What I have not yet shared with you is that Avis was a junior world golfer at age ten. She has been playing golf since age five and went on to play in the LPGA, but had to give up her dream because of finances. She is one of only four African American women who played on tour. All her life she has practiced hard and has had determination, mental toughness, discipline, and humility. Now Avis *and her family run a golf program for kids in the San Diego schools and a junior program to help teens learn life lessons on and off the golf course. She plans to obtain her PGA card and play in the LPGA again.*

You go, girl!

Be Positive

Rise, shine, succeed, and face your future. You must press on and push forward toward your destiny.

Be Fruitful

BREAKFAST: Shakeology Breakfast at Hazel's

Combine 1 packet of Chocolate Shakeology mix (or 6 ounces of any low-sugar protein powder), 1 teaspoon hazelnut extract, 1 cup water, and ice to taste (add more ice for a thicker shake). Blend until creamy.

> 152 calories, 17 grams protein, 20 grams carbohydrate,
> 1 gram fat, 3 grams fiber

SNACK: Nachos

Slice open 1 small (4-inch diameter) whole-wheat pita and brush very lightly with ⅛ teaspoon extra-virgin olive oil. Cut into triangular wedges. Sprinkle 3 teaspoons low-fat, low-sodium cheddar cheese evenly over pita wedges. Season with a pinch (⅛ teaspoon) of dried oregano. Heat under broiler until cheese is melted. Add a slice of jalapeño, if desired. Enjoy with an 8-ounce glass of water.

> 120 calories, 8 grams protein, 16 grams carbohydrate,
> 3 grams fat, 2 grams fiber

LUNCH: Egg Salad Sandwich

Blend 2 teaspoons low-fat mayonnaise, ⅛ teaspoon garlic powder, ⅛ teaspoon celery seed, and ⅛ teaspoon dried oregano in a large bowl. Season to taste with your favorite salt-free seasoning. Add 1 large hard-boiled egg, chopped; the egg white from 1 hard-boiled egg, chopped; and ¼ cup fresh diced celery. Mix. Spoon egg salad between bread slices. Enjoy with a small (4 ounces) glass of fat-free milk.

> 310 calories, 22 grams protein, 32 grams carbohydrate,
> 10 grams fat, 4 grams fiber

SNACK: Pesto-Artichoke Chicken Wrap

Shred 2 tablespoons cooked chicken. In a small bowl, mix together shredded chicken, 2½ teaspoons fresh, cooked, or canned artichoke hearts, coarsely chopped, and ½ teaspoon fresh chopped scallions. Set aside. Spread ½ teaspoon pesto sauce on a 6-inch low-carb flour tortilla. Arrange chicken mix with a piece of pimento on top. Roll up tortilla; heat if desired. Enjoy with a glass of water.

> 120 calories, 9 grams protein, 13 grams carbohydrate,
> 3.5 grams fat, 8 grams fiber

DINNER: Mediterranean Cod

In a small bowl, combine ¾ cup chopped tomatoes, 2 teaspoons chopped green onions, 2 teaspoons chopped basil, 6 chopped black olives, ⅛ teaspoon garlic powder, 2 teaspoons extra-virgin olive oil, 1½ teaspoons lemon juice, and 1 tablespoon balsamic vinegar. Let stand at room temperature. Preheat oven to 425°F. Lightly coat a shallow baking dish with nonstick cooking spray. Rinse the fish and pat dry with a paper towel. Place fish in prepared baking dish. Drizzle with 1½ teaspoons lemon juice and top with tomato mixture. Bake until just cooked through, approximately 10 to 12 minutes, or until fish flakes easily with a fork.

Quick and Easy Couscous

Prepare couscous per package directions. Portion out ⅔ cup. Drizzle with ¾ teaspoon olive oil and top with ½ teaspoon fresh chopped parsley.

Dessert: Honeydew and Grapes

Enjoy ¾ cup honeydew melon balls and ⅓ cup fresh grapes (any color) for dessert.

> 580 calories, 42 grams protein, 59 grams carbohydrate,
> 19 grams fat, 5 grams fiber

Be Joyful

SONG OF THE DAY: "Takin' Care of Business" by Bachman-Turner Overdrive

Be Fit

WARM-UP: 3–5 minutes
CARDIO: Butt-Kicking
STRENGTH TRAINING: 10–20 minutes
STRETCH: 3–5 minutes

Butt-Kicking Workout

Front Jab and Jump

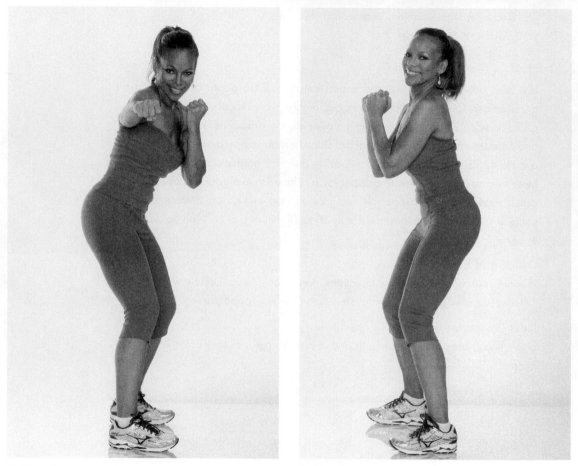

Position A

Position B

Face your left side, standing tall with your feet hip-width apart and your arms bent at chest level. Extend your right arm forward, then pull your fist back in (front jab), and perform three jabs (Position A). Then turn to the right by doing three jumps with your feet remaining hip-width apart. Now you are facing the opposite direction (Position B). Perform three front jabs with your left arm followed by three jumps with your feet hip-width apart to turn back. Perform front-jab-jump series 6–10 times, alternating from side to side.

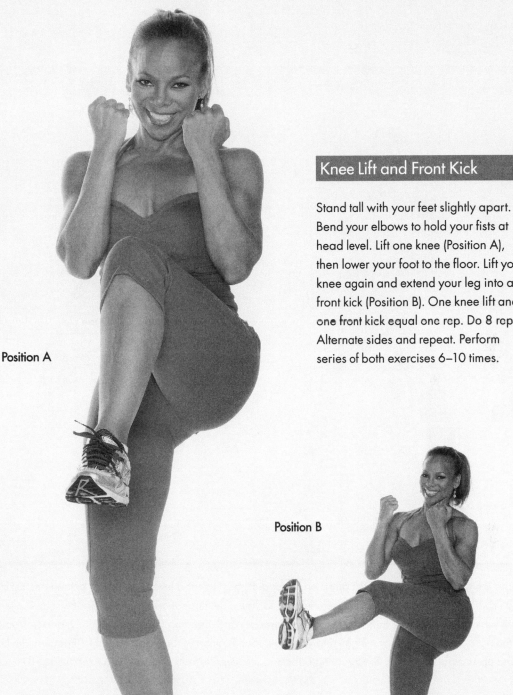

Position A

Knee Lift and Front Kick

Stand tall with your feet slightly apart. Bend your elbows to hold your fists at head level. Lift one knee (Position A), then lower your foot to the floor. Lift your knee again and extend your leg into a front kick (Position B). One knee lift and one front kick equal one rep. Do 8 reps. Alternate sides and repeat. Perform series of both exercises 6–10 times.

Position B

Front Jabs and Bob and Weave

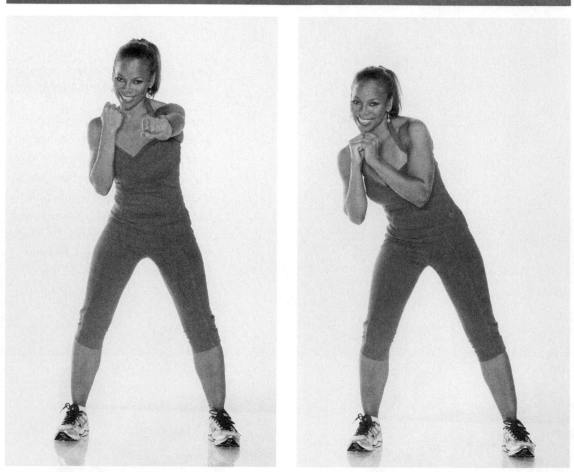

Position A   **Position B**

Stand tall with your feet hip-width apart and your arms bent at chest level. Make fists, extend one fist forward in a jab (Position A), then bring your elbow back to your side. Repeat on the other side. Perform 8 alternating front jabs. Then hold your hands at chest level, lean forward, bending your knees slightly, and shift your torso to the right, distributing your weight onto your right foot (Position B). Stand up straight. Repeat on the left, then stand up straight again. Do 8 alternating bobs and weaves. Perform series of both exercises 6–10 times.

Side Kicks with Side Crunch

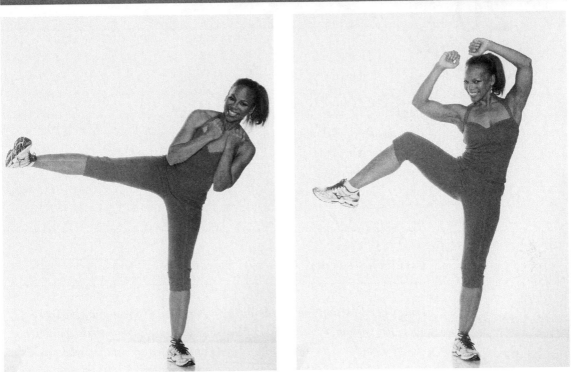

Position A

Position B

Stand tall and face forward with your elbows bent and your fists at chest level. Lean to one side and kick out to the opposite side (Position A). Repeat on the opposite side. Do 8 reps. Then with your elbows bent and held at head level, bend your torso to the side, bringing your knee up and your arms down (Position B). Repeat on the opposite side. Do 8 reps again. Perform series of both exercises 6–10 times.

REPEAT CIRCUIT 1–3 TIMES.

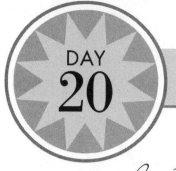

DAY 20

Daily Spread

Be Faithful

*I can do all things through Christ
which strengthens me.*

—PHILIPPIANS 4:13

Be Grateful

CHERYL'S STORY

I met Cheryl "Action" Jackson through my best friend. The minute she spoke about her passion, I could feel her heart and determination to make a difference. Her food pantry is named Minnie's Food Pantry after her mother, who was the wife of a pastor and committed her life to serving others. Cheryl grew up seeing her parents help people at church and at their home. Later in life, Cheryl was the one who needed help. She and her husband struggled to make ends meet for their family of four. She applied for food stamps but was denied and just given a bag of food to take home. Eventually, she and her husband worked many jobs to get the family financially stable.

Cheryl was then faced with the death of her father. It was during this time that her calling became very clear: help feed those in need. She opened Minnie's Pantry to feed the hungry. When people come into her pantry, they walk the red carpet with a cart to pick up food and receive love and nurturing from Cheryl. Music plays, people sing, and healthy kids' bags are handed out. Cheryl shares her story with them because she was once in their shoes. She feels their pain, and a connection is made. When she didn't have rent money to keep the pantry open, she left the building to figure out how she could get the money. She asked God to show her a sign that it was going to all work out. Her assistant called and told her to come to the pantry right away because a couple of kids were there with signs that read, "When I was hungry, you fed me." They raised $2,135 selling M&Ms

to give back to the person who had helped them—Cheryl. The money covered the rent and kept the pantry doors open.

So far, Minnie's Food Pantry has helped over 93,000 people and served 1.3 million pounds of food. Donations of food and money keep the pantry going. She recently started taking food to day laborers who show up at various sites in hopes of getting a job for the day. Thanks to Cheryl, they at least get a meal. In the works is her own TV show, Action Jackson Is Hungry. She wants to raise awareness about hunger and hopes to inspire others to take action. She started with a heart to serve by giving away food from her own pantry. Cheryl says she always keeps in mind what Oprah shared with her, "Do that what you do and do it as if you were not paid to do it."

Be Positive

Make an attitude adjustment.
Think it, believe it, speak it.

Be Fruitful

BREAKFAST: Corned Beef Hash

Heat 1¾ teaspoons canola oil over medium-high heat. Dice 4 ounces deli-sliced corned beef. Sauté 3 tablespoons chopped onions and 2 tablespoons chopped red bell peppers in skillet until tender. Add corned beef and ⅔ cup diced potatoes and cook until potatoes are soft and browned. Serve 6 ounces plain nonfat yogurt topped with ⅔ cup fresh strawberries on the side. Enjoy breakfast with a cup of coffee or tea or other calorie-free beverage.

Tip: Soak corned beef in water and wring out prior to cooking to reduce sodium content.

390 calories, 28 grams protein, 44 grams carbohydrate,
14 grams fat, 5 grams fiber

SNACK: Pumpkin Seeds

Enjoy 2½ teaspoons pumpkin seeds and a small (4 ounces) glass of orange juice for this quick, crunchy snack.

90 calories, 3 grams protein, 14 grams carbohydrate,
3.5 grams fat, <1 gram fiber

LUNCH: Orange Sunshine Shake

Blend 1 packet of Tropical Strawberry Shakeology mix (or 6 ounces of any low-sugar protein powder), ½ cup 100% orange juice, 1 cup water, and ice to taste (add more ice for a thicker shake).

> 215 calories, 16 grams protein, 33 grams carbohydrate,
> 1.25 grams fat, 3 grams fiber

SNACK: Chicken Salad

Shred 2½ tablespoons cooked chicken breast. Mix chicken with 1 teaspoon low-fat mayonnaise and a dash (⅛ teaspoon) of dried dill weed. Serve with (or on) 1 piece thin-sliced whole-wheat bread. Enjoy with an 8-ounce glass of water.

> 120 calories, 9 grams protein, 11 grams carbohydrate,
> 3.5 grams fat, 2 grams fiber

DINNER: Herbed Shrimp Sauté

In a medium bowl, toss 6¼ ounces uncooked shrimp with 1 teaspoon chopped garlic, 1 teaspoon fresh chopped parsley, 1 teaspoon fresh rosemary, ¼ teaspoon ground thyme, and ½ teaspoon extra-virgin olive oil; set aside for 15 minutes. Place ½ teaspoon extra-virgin olive oil in a medium nonstick skillet and heat over medium-high heat. Add the shrimp and sauce. Sauté, stirring constantly, until the shrimp are cooked through, about 3 to 5 minutes. Add 1 teaspoon lemon juice and 2 tablespoons fat-free, low-sodium chicken broth to the skillet, scraping up any browned bits on the bottom of the skillet. Cook over medium-high heat, stirring frequently, until reduced by half. Add 1 teaspoon canola-based, trans-fat-free margarine and continue to cook until melted. Pour sauce over shrimp and ⅓ cup rice. Season with ⅛ teaspoon black pepper and serve hot.

Zucchini

Heat ½ teaspoon extra-virgin olive oil over medium flame. Add 1⅔ cup fresh sliced zucchini and sauté until tender. Season with salt and black pepper to taste.

Macaroni Pasta and Vegetable Salad

Toss ⅓ cup cooked macaroni noodles with 2 tablespoons reduced-fat (⅓ less) Italian salad dressing, 1½ tablespoons balsamic vinegar, 2 tablespoons sliced mushrooms, 2 tablespoons chopped green bell pepper, and 5 cherry tomatoes.

Dessert: Sugar-Free Fudge Bar and Berries

Enjoy 1 sugar-free fudge bar (45 calories) with ¾ cup raspberries.

> 600 calories, 46 grams protein, 56 grams carbohydrate,
> 22 grams fat, 11 grams fiber

Be Joyful

SONG OF THE DAY: "Show Me the Way" by Peter Frampton

Be Fit

WARM-UP: 3–4 minutes

CARDIO: 30–60 minutes

STRENGTH TRAINING: Game Time

STRETCH: 3–5 minutes

Game Time Workout

Inner-Thigh Leg Lift

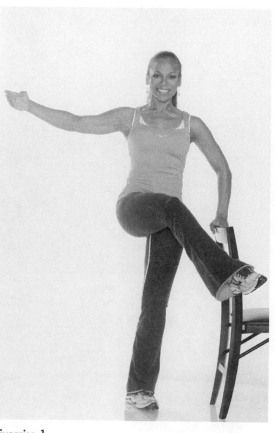

Outer-Thigh Leg Lift

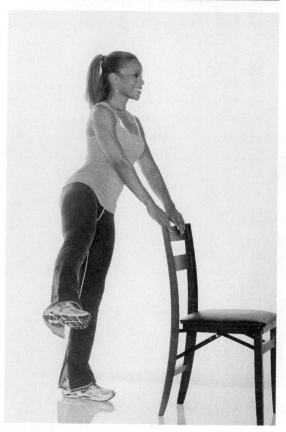

Exercise 1

Stand tall with your feet hip-width apart. Let one hand rest on a chair with your other arm extended to the side at shoulder height. Bring your outside leg up and across your body, then lower it back to the starting position. Do 16 reps. On the last rep, hold your leg up for 32 counts. Return to the starting position. Turn around, put your other hand on the chair, and repeat.

Exercise 2

Stand tall with your feet hip-width apart. Face a chair with your hands resting on the chair back. Lift one leg out to the side, then return to the starting position. Do 16 reps, on the last rep holding your leg up for 32 counts. Then return to the starting position. Repeat on the other side.

Reverse Plank

Exercise 3

Sit on the edge of a chair, holding on to the sides of the chair. Straighten your legs in front of you with your feet together and flat on the floor. Straighten your arms and lift your hips until your body forms a straight line from head to toe. Hold for a count of three, and then lower yourself back down to the chair. Perform 16 reps.

Seated Crunch

Exercise 4

Sit on the edge of a chair, holding on to the sides of the chair or the armrests. Lean back 45 degrees, lift your feet, and contract your abs, bringing your knees to your chest. Hold for 5 counts, then touch your feet to the ground and repeat. Perform 16 reps.

Squat Dips

Exercise 5

Stand 2 feet from a sturdy chair with your feet hip-width apart and your hands on your hips. Lift one leg behind you and place your foot on the seat of the chair. Bend your knee and lower yourself into a single-leg lunge, with the front knee over your heel and the back knee bent. Straighten your front leg and return to the starting position. Perform 16 reps, then switch legs and repeat.

Seated Leg Extension

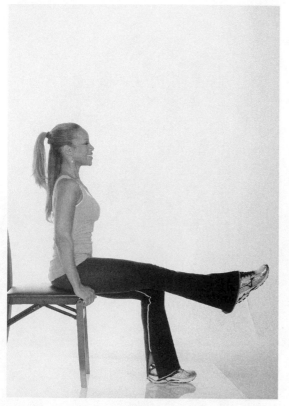

Chair Push-Up

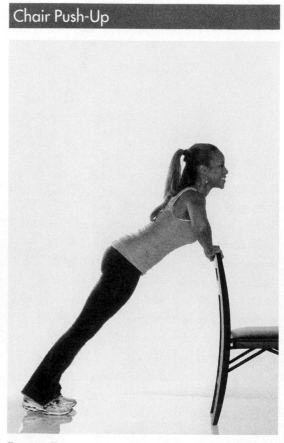

Exercise 6

Sit tall on the edge of a chair, knees bent, feet flat on the floor, and hands resting beside your buttocks. Extend your right leg forward and hold for 8 counts, then lower your foot back to the floor. Lengthen your left leg and hold for 8 counts, then lower it to the floor. Alternate sides. Perform 16 reps.

Exercise 7

Stand tall several feet behind a sturdy chair, with your arms straight, your feet hip-width apart, and your hands placed on the back of the chair. Bend your arms and lower your chest toward the chair. Straighten your arms and return to the starting position. Perform 16 reps.

Single-Leg Bridge

Exercise 8

Lie on your back on the floor or a mat with your legs extended and your heels resting on the seat of a chair. Rest your arms on the floor with your palms down. Lift one leg straight up as you contract your buttocks and lift your hips. Lower yourself back to the starting position. Do 16 reps. Hold your last rep for 32 counts, then return to the starting position. Switch legs and repeat.

REPEAT CIRCUIT 1–3 TIMES.

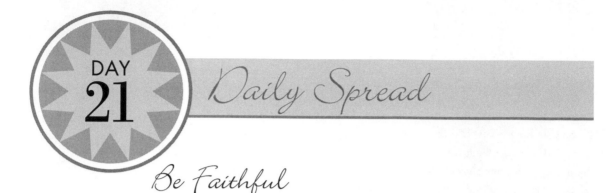

Be Faithful

*Let us not become weary in doing good,
for at the proper time we will reap a
harvest if we do not give up.*
—GALATIANS 6:9

Be Grateful

DR. JILL'S STORY

For over twenty years, Dr. Jill has practiced helping her patients integrate all aspects of health and wellness so they can live optimal lives. She shows them how to take care of themselves when they aren't well and how to heal their bodies to return to a state of well-being. She feels that many of her female patients experience emotions that affect them physically. Because women feel with their hearts, when our hearts are broken we experience physical manifestations of that heartbreak. Therefore, our physical problems can be directly related to emotional problems. As women, we take care of everyone else and forget to take care of ourselves; we run ourselves into the ground trying to do it all. Dr. Jill, like myself, tries to help women connect the dots. Your well-being is based upon your overall health—mental, emotional, physical, and spiritual.

Dr. Jill creates a safe place where her patients can share what they feel. She addresses their concerns and recommends the best solutions. Her goal is to build trust so she can better serve her patients. She believes that medicine is ministry. Once upon a time, when she was an intern working thirty-six-hour shifts, a distraught woman came to the emergency room in the middle of the night. Dr. Jill spent time trying to calm her down. Although she wasn't being medically treated, the same woman showed up on many subsequent nights wanting to talk to Dr. Jill. Eventually Dr. Jill discovered that the woman's husband had recently died and she couldn't deal with being alone. Dr. Jill was able to get her grief therapy and to work with her family to better support her.

Dr. Jill walks the walk when it comes to her medical ministry. She shares her struggles and challenges with her patients and lets them know that she is their health partner. She is not afraid to speak about her faith or offer prayer. She is not afraid to cry. She is not afraid to give a hug. She keeps it real and gives the real deal.

A patient once shared her food diary with Dr. Jill, and it was horrific. When Dr. Jill explained the importance of baking or grilling fish and chicken, her patient said, "I only know how to fry meat." Dr. Jill showed her how to cook healthier, including how to turn her deep fryer into a steamer to cook vegetables.

I admire the excellent work and dedication of Dr. Jill. She serves as a great role model for other physicians.

Doc, you rock!

Be Positive

Fill your heart with joy and demonstrate love in everything
you say and do. Stay positive and be kind.

Be Fruitful

BREAKFAST: Bacon-Egg Sandwich

Cut 1 whole-wheat English muffin in half and spread both halves evenly with 2 teaspoons canola-based trans-fat-free margarine. Cook ½ cup egg substitute over medium-high heat in a skillet lightly coated with cooking spray. Heat 1 ounce Canadian bacon briefly on both sides in a small skillet. Remove egg from heat and place on bottom half of the English muffin. Top with Canadian bacon and other half of muffin. Enjoy with ½ cup blueberries on the side and a cup of coffee or tea.

> 390 calories, 27 grams protein, 39 grams carbohydrate,
> 15 grams fat, 6 grams fiber

SNACK: Ham-Wrapped Dates

Cut 1½ ounces low-sodium, thinly sliced ham into 2 strips. Wrap ham strips around 2 whole dates and enjoy with an 8-ounce glass of water.

> 120 calories, 10 grams protein, 13 grams carbohydrate,
> 3.5 grams fat, 1 gram fiber

LUNCH: Chocolate Twilight Shake

Blend 1 packet of Chocolate Shakeology mix (or 6 ounces of any low-sugar protein powder), 1 teaspoon vanilla extract, 1 cup water, and ice to taste (add more ice for a thicker shake).

144 calories, 17 grams protein, 18 grams carbohydrate, 1 gram fat, 3 grams fiber

SNACK: Soy Nuts and Raisins

Enjoy 1½ tablespoons dry-roasted, unsalted soy beans and 2 teaspoons raisins.

100 calories, 6 grams protein, 11 grams carbohydrate, 4 grams fat, 3 grams fiber

DINNER: Parmesan-Dijon Chicken

Preheat oven to 375°F. Mix 1½ tablespoons seasoned bread crumbs and 1 tablespoon fat-free Parmesan cheese and spread out on a plate. Melt 1 teaspoon low-fat buttery spread and combine with ½ teaspoon Dijon mustard in a shallow dish. Dip 6 ounces of boneless, skinless chicken breast into spread mixture, then coat with bread crumb mixture. Place in baking dish. Dot with 1⅓ tablespoons low-fat buttery spread. Bake uncovered 20 to 25 minutes, turning once, or until chicken is no longer pink inside.

Peas and Carrots

Heat ½ cup frozen peas and carrots in a small saucepan or in the microwave per package directions. Top with ¾ teaspoon low-fat buttery spread.

Garlic Bread

Combine 1 teaspoon low-fat buttery spread and ¼ teaspoon chopped garlic in a small saucepan. Stir until melted. Brush onto ½ medium whole-wheat hoagie roll. Sprinkle with ¼ teaspoon dried parsley. Place on baking sheet and broil until golden.

Desert: Chocolate-and-Nut-Coated Banana

Coat ½ small banana with 1½ tablespoons fat-free light chocolate syrup. Sprinkle with 1 teaspoon chopped pecans. Place in refrigerator or freezer to set. Enjoy for dessert.

600 calories, 45 grams protein, 61 grams carbohydrate, 20 grams fat, 8 grams fiber

Be Joyful

SONG OF THE DAY: "Closer" by Ne-Yo

Be Fit

Weekly Fitness Diary

_____

_____

_____

_____

_____

_____

_____

_____

_____

_____

_____

_____

_____

_____

_____

_____

_____

_____

_____

_____

_____

_____

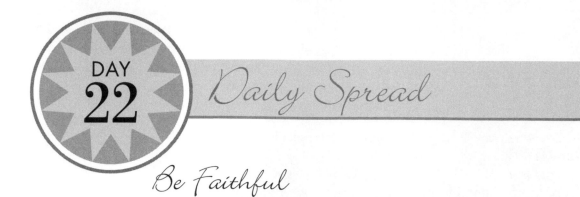

22

Daily Spread

Be Faithful

*For God has not given us the spirit of fear; but of
power, and of love, and of a sound mind.*
—2 TIMOTHY 1:7

Be Grateful

SARAH'S STORY

I met Sarah while teaching at my friend Pat's Treasure You retreat. We spoke right
after my class, and I realized that she was the amazing woman that my friend
had been telling me about. A year before, I had played golf with Sarah's husband,
who had introduced me to her healthy foods product line. Sarah had been a
mover and shaker, a CEO for major corporations, but decided to turn down a
great job opportunity to launch a healthy food company called Hail Merry. Sarah
said she took a leap of faith because she had learned she had diabetes. By divine
intervention, she partnered with Susan O'Brien and became the CEO of a company
that made healthy foods for everyone, including those with diabetes.

In two and a half years Hail Merry went from being distributed in eight stores
to a reach of over six hundred stores with fifteen products. What Sarah had done
for other companies, she was now doing for her own, and she was enjoying sweet
success. Yes, she is driven about her work, but her passion to make a difference is
her greatest asset. Sarah joined forces with Marian Wright Edelman, president
of the Children's Defense Fund, to work with her program Beat the Odds, which
provides resources for students to receive a good education. Sarah's passion to
educate children started with her late father, who was a school principal, and
her mother, who was a teacher. Last year the program awarded three students
$20,000 in scholarship funds for the college of their choice.

The first recipient of the scholarship was Prentice Richmond. Sarah and
those she worked with had no idea that this young man was homeless when he
received the award, but soon she made a way and provided shelter for him in

the pool cabana where Susan had started Hail Merry Foods. Prentice had been homeless since ninth grade, but he excelled in school; he earned great grades, was the captain of the football team, and served as volunteer coach for Midnight Basketball. He now attends the University of Texas A&M Commerce and works as a teacher for at-risk kids. In addition to Prentice, six others have been awarded the scholarship and over a hundred have received a separate scholarship, Emerald Eagles, which includes free tuition, room, and board. I'm inspired and empowered by Sarah, who uses the gifts God has given her to be a beacon of light and to help others fulfill their purpose in life. She is an example of my motto, "Live to give."

Be Positive

When it seems as though you're up against a wall, refocus and rebuild, and know in your heart that you can turn to a power greater than you!

Be Fruitful

BREAKFAST: Almond Paradise Shake

Combine 1 packet of Tropical Strawberry Shakeology mix (or 6 ounces of any low-sugar protein powder), 1 cup unsweetened almond milk, 1 teaspoon natural almond butter, 1 cup water, and ice to taste (add more ice for a thicker shake). Blend until creamy.

232.5 calories, 17.5 grams protein, 23 grams carbohydrate, 6.7 grams fat, 3 grams fiber

SNACK: Hard-Boiled Egg

Enjoy a 1 large hard-boiled egg and half a small banana for this quick snack.

120 calories, 7 grams protein, 12 grams carbohydrate, 5 grams fat, 1 gram fiber

LUNCH: Philly Cheesesteak Sandwich

Preheat oven to 400°F. In a small bowl, combine 2 teaspoons low-fat mayonnaise and ¼ teaspoon chopped garlic. Cover and refrigerate. Slice 2½ ounces beef sirloin into thin strips. Spray a skillet with nonstick cooking spray; heat on medium-high. Sauté beef until lightly browned. Stir in ⅓ cup sliced green bell pepper and ¼ cup chopped onion. Sauté vegetables until tender and remove from heat. Spread hot dog bun with garlic mayonnaise and fill with beef mixture. Top with 1 tablespoon shredded part-skim mozzarella and ¼ teaspoon dried oregano. Heat sandwich in preheated oven until cheese is melted. Enjoy with your favorite calorie-free beverage.

280 calories, 22 grams protein, 27 grams carbohydrate,
9 grams fat, 2 grams fiber

SNACK: Cottage Cheese and Strawberries

Top ⅓ cup low-fat (1%) cottage cheese with 6 whole fresh strawberries and 1½ tablespoons chopped pecans. Enjoy with an 8-ounce glass of water.

110 calories, 9 grams protein, 13 grams carbohydrate,
4 grams fat, 2 grams fiber

DINNER: Dilled Salmon

Preheat grill or broiler. Prepare dill sauce by combining ½ teaspoon fresh dill, ⅛ teaspoon black pepper, 1½ teaspoons mustard (any flavor), 1½ teaspoons white rice vinegar, 2 tablespoons fat-free sour cream, and ½ tablespoon chopped green onion. Refrigerate until ready to serve. Brush 6 ounces fresh wild Alaskan or Washington salmon with 1½ teaspoons extra-virgin olive oil and grill over hot coals (or broil) for 5 to 8 minutes per side, depending on thickness, or until fish flakes easily with fork. Serve topped with dill sauce.

Roasted Brussels Sprouts

Preheat oven to 400°F. Coat a baking sheet with cooking spray. Toss ¾ cup fresh brussels sprouts with ½ teaspoon extra-virgin olive oil and ⅛ teaspoon black pepper. Place on baking sheet and roast for 30 to 45 minutes. Shake pan every 5 to 10 minutes for even browning.

White Rice

Prepare ⅓ cup instant white rice per package directions. Top with 1½ teaspoons low-fat buttery spread and enjoy.

Kiwi and Strawberry Dessert

Serve 2 peeled and sliced kiwis with ¼ cup fresh sliced strawberries for a refreshing dessert.

580 calories, 42 grams protein, 60 grams carbohydrate,
20 grams fat, 8 grams fiber

Be Joyful

SONG OF THE DAY: "Rhythm Is Gonna Get You" by Gloria Estefan

Be Fit

WARM-UP: 3–5 minutes

CARDIO: 30–60 minutes

STRENGTH TRAINING: Red Carpet

STRETCH: 3–5 minutes

Red Carpet Workout

Dead Lift and Bent-Over Row

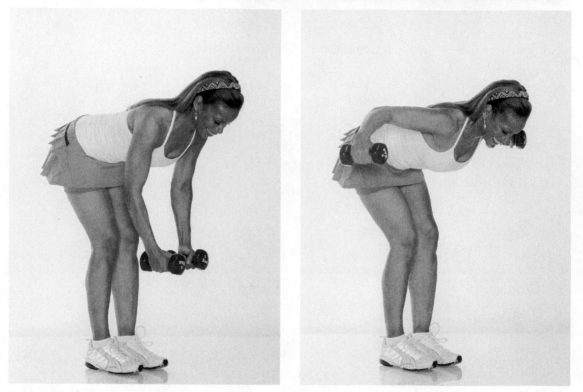

Position A　　　　　　　　　　　　　　　　　　　　　　　　**Position B**

Stand tall with feet hip-width apart, holding weights in your hands. Hold your arms in front of you at hip level with your palms facing inward. Bend forward at your hips, keeping your back parallel to the floor and letting your arms hang down (Position A). Extend your arms up and out to your sides (Position B). Return to the standing position and lower the weights to the front of your hips. Perform 16 reps.

Lunge and Bicep Curl

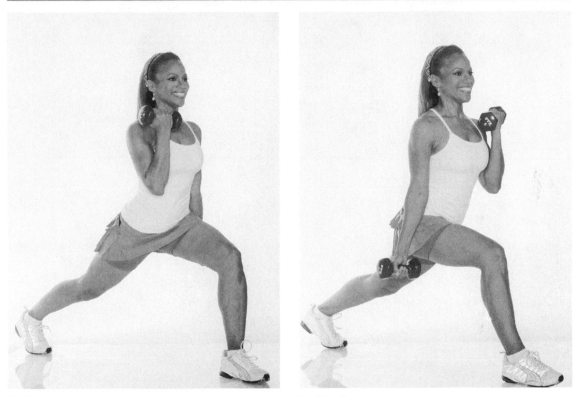

Position A

Position B

Start in a forward lunge with your left foot forward, holding weights in your hands and keeping your arms at your sides. Lift the weight in your right hand to shoulder level (Position A), then straighten to a standing position while bringing the weight back down to your side. Come into a forward lunge with your right foot forward, while simultaneously lifting the weight in your left hand to your shoulder (Position B). Straighten to a standing position while bringing the weight back down to your side. Perform 16 reps. On the last rep, pulse in lunge position and do small alternating bicep curls. (The focus of the lunge is on lifting up, instead of like in a traditional lunge, which focuses on a downward movement.)

Chest Press

Start in a standing position with your feet more than shoulder-width apart, weights in both hands, arms bent and held out to the sides at chest level, and palms facing forward (Position A). Lower into a plié position, while bringing the weights together in front of your chest (Position B). Push up and return to the starting position. Perform 16 reps.

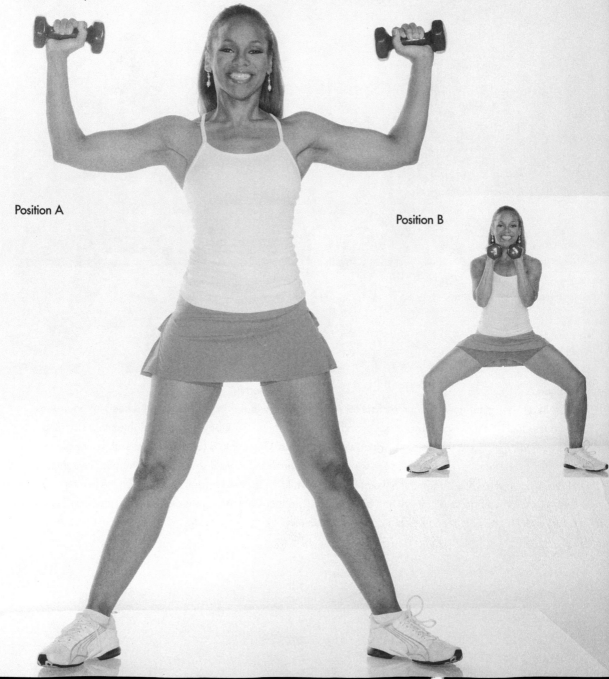

Position A

Position B

Bend and Heel Lift

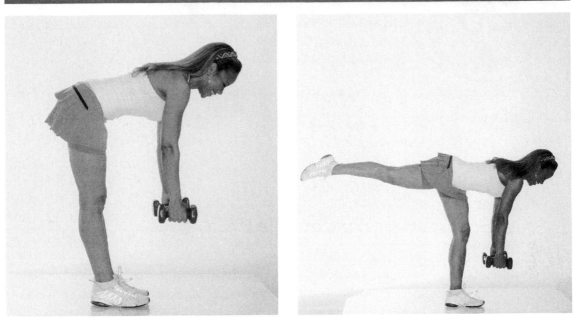

Position A   Position B

Start in a standing position with weights in your hands. Bend at your waist, allowing your arms to hang down in front, palms facing inward (Position A). Raise your right leg straight behind you (Position B). Lower your leg to the floor. Raise your left leg straight behind you. Perform 16 reps.

REPEAT CIRCUIT 1–3 TIMES.

Be Faithful

Be joyful in hope, patient in affliction, faithful in prayer.
—ROMANS 12:12

Be Grateful

CELEBRATING OUR DIFFERENCES

As I read a story in the Washington Times *about Heather Greenwood and her family, I thought about my godson and the race problems we still face as a nation. Years ago, when my godson, Ricardo, was in grade school, he came home one day perplexed because he was asked, "What color are you?" He responded by saying that he was "brown," adding, "Can't they see?" Twenty-five years later, Heather's daughter Sophia responds when asked what race she is, "Tan!" The second grader goes on to ask, "Can't you tell by just looking?"*

My friend Michelle has an African father and a Caucasian mother. Her husband, Aaron, is Caucasian. Although at home they are color-blind, the minute they leave home, people stare, make rude comments, and tell offensive jokes. One day at the checkout stand, a Caucasian woman noticed Michelle and her child, who has light skin, blond curls, and blue eyes. The woman said, "It's not possible—you are so dark!" Shaken by this woman's statement, Michelle responded, "How come? That's the way God made us." We are making strides, but we must work harder to see through a lens that is color-blind. Instead of dividing ourselves, we must unite and live in the spirit of Martin Luther King's dream that "one day children will live in a nation where they will be judged not by the color of their skin but by the content of their character."

I have traveled around the world learning about people and cultures. I speak about health and insist that health has no color. It does not matter what shape, size, age, color, or nationality we are; we all should take the best care of our bodies, which are our temples. Unfortunately, race and economic factors contribute to the health disparities in this country. In the Bible it says to love thy neighbor—and it does not specify our white, black, brown, or tan neighbor. If someone is about to bless you, does it matter what color he or she is? If someone is in need of an organ, does it matter the color of the organ donor, as long as it's a match? If there is a life-and-death situation, our natural instincts take over to help save a life regardless of the person's color.

Let's celebrate our individuality and embrace our differences. Let's flow in God's sea of love, which is colorful, compassionate, and contagious!

Be Positive

Don't judge yourself based on external factors and the opinions of the outside world. Motivation comes from within, so start planting positive seeds and reap a harvest of hope!

Be Fruitful

BREAKFAST: Oat Bran Cereal with Raspberries

Combine ⅓ cup dry oat bran cereal and 8 ounces fat-free milk into a bowl; heat according to package directions. Stir in ¼ cup raspberries and 1 teaspoon roasted coarsely chopped almonds. Prepare 2 turkey breakfast sausage links per package directions and serve on the side. Enjoy with a cup of coffee or tea, or another calorie-free beverage.

> 400 calories, 29 grams protein, 41 grams carbohydrate,
> 14 grams fat, 7 grams fiber

SNACK: Salmon Salad on Crispbread

Wash ¼ medium tomato and peel ¼ cucumber; slice thinly. Drain 1 ounce salmon (canned in water) and combine with 1 teaspoon low-fat mayonnaise and ½ teaspoon Dijon mustard in a small bowl. Spread salmon salad onto 2 low-sodium crispbread crackers; top with tomato and cucumber slices. Enjoy with a glass of water.

> 120 calories, 8 grams protein, 15 grams carbohydrate,
> 3.5 grams fat, 3 grams fiber

LUNCH: Strawberry Tango Shake

Blend 1 packet of Greenberry Shakeology mix (or 6 ounces of any low-sugar protein powder), ½ cup strawberries, ½ cup mango, 1 cup water, and ice to taste (add more ice for a thicker shake).

> 230 calories, 16 grams protein, 57 grams carbohydrate,
> 0.5 grams fat, 3 grams fiber

SNACK: Beef Jerky

Enjoy ¾ ounce California-style, teriyaki-flavored beef jerky, 2 whole-wheat crackers, and an 8-ounce glass of water for this simple snack.

> 130 calories, 11 grams protein, 15 grams carbohydrate,
> 3.5 grams fat, 2 grams fiber

DINNER: Stuffed Green Pepper

Preheat oven to 350°F. Cut a slice from the top of 1 large green bell pepper; remove seeds and membrane. Cook pepper shell in boiling water for 5 minutes. Drain well. Heat 1½ teaspoons extra-virgin olive oil in a medium skillet over medium-high heat; sauté ¼ cup chopped onion and ½ cup diced fresh celery in 2 tablespoons fat-free, low-sodium chicken broth until tender. Remove mixture and set aside. In the same skillet, brown and drain 5 ounces lean (5% fat) ground beef. Add vegetable mixture back into the skillet with meat, stirring to combine, and turn off heat. Stir in 2 tablespoons liquid egg substitute, 1 teaspoon fresh chopped parsley, ⅛ teaspoon black pepper, and ⅛ teaspoon dried basil. Fill pepper shell with meat mixture and place in a baking dish lightly coated with nonstick cooking spray. Pour hot water to a depth of ¼ inch around pepper. Bake 30 minutes.

Wild Rice

Prepare wild rice per package directions. Serve ⅔ cup of rice topped with 2 teaspoons low-fat buttery spread with dinner.

Frozen Yogurt and Berries

Enjoy ¼ cup nonfat, sugar-free, chocolate frozen yogurt topped with ⅔ cup blackberries and 1 teaspoon fat-free light chocolate syrup.

> 580 calories, 45 grams protein, 56 grams carbohydrate,
> 20 grams fat, 11 grams fiber

Be Joyful

SONG OF THE DAY: "You Belong with Me" by Taylor Swift

Be Fit

WARM-UP: 3–5 minutes

CARDIO: 30–60 minutes

STRENGTH TRAINING: Trim, Toned, and Tight

STRETCH: 3–5 minutes

Trim, Toned, and Tight Workout

Lunge and Tricep Overhead

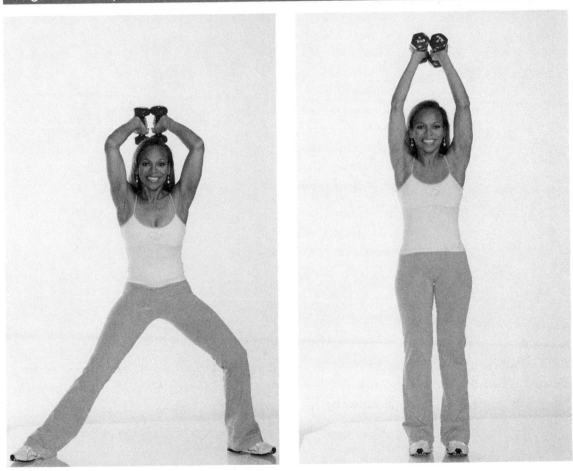

Position A

Position B

Start in a side lunge position with your arms bent, elbows next to your ears, and hands holding weights behind your head (Position A). Extend your arms upward, while coming to a standing position (Position B). Repeat on the opposite side. Do 15 reps.

Squat and Bicep Curl with Front Kick

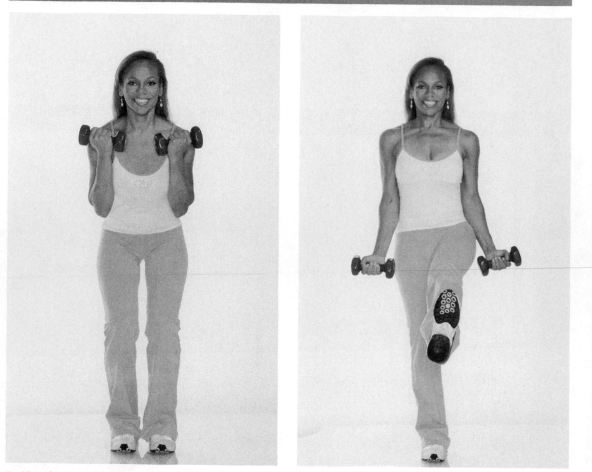

Position A

Position B

Stand tall with your feet slightly apart, holding weights with your arms at your sides. Squat down while lifting the weights toward your shoulders (Position A), then stand up and kick one leg in front of you while lowering the weights to your sides (Position B). Repeat on the other side. Perform 15 reps.

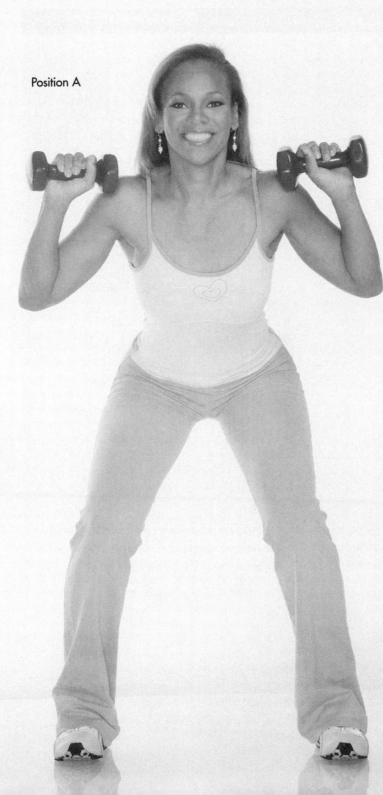

Position A

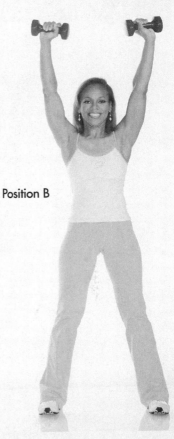

Position B

Squat and Shoulder Press

Stand tall with your feet more than hip-width apart and your elbows bent, holding weights in your hands at shoulder level with your palms facing forward (Position A). Push up and extend your arms above your head (Position B). Return to the start position. Perform 15 reps.

Tricep Kickback and Leg Lift

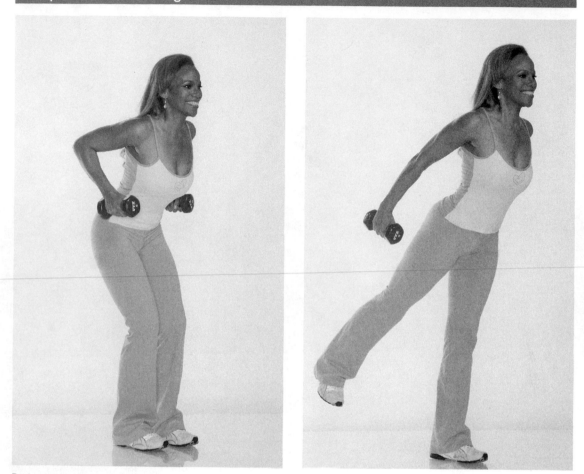

Position A

Position B

Start with your feet hip-width apart in a semi-squat position with your elbows pointing back and weights in your hands (Position A). Straighten up and lift one leg behind you as you extend your arms back (Position B). Lower your leg and return to the starting position. Repeat on the opposite side. Perform 15 reps.

REPEAT CIRCUIT 1–3 TIMES.

Be Faithful

Train up a child in the way he should go:
and when he is old, he will not depart from it.
—PROVERBS 22:6

Be Grateful

TAYLOR'S STORY

Taylor, my friend's son, has so much heart to give. He will soon graduate with
a degree in biology. Originally, he wanted to become a doctor so he could help
people. Now he has decided to become a nurse and earn an MBA in business
administration.

Recently, Taylor was with his mom at Minnie's Food Pantry, which feeds
thousands of people in need. A group of women, myself included, were there to
learn about this company and offer assistance. Not knowing Taylor's goal at
the time, I asked his mom, Cherice, "How did you get your son to join us this
afternoon?" She said, "He wanted to come and learn about how Cheryl runs
her nonprofit company." I was surprised but also filled with hope that this young
man, age twenty-one, was all about helping others.

The year before, Taylor had taken a trip to Honduras for two weeks to do
missionary work. He served at a community center, a school, and a shelter. At the
shelter he met teenage mothers who had come to learn life and job skills. He spoke
with the young ladies, cuddled their babies, and prayed with them. Although
the girls didn't speak English, they belted out every word of Justin Bieber's songs
when Taylor played them. When it was time for him to leave, a thirteen-year-
old mom said to him, "You are a good person, and one day you are going to be a
good father."

Before he left for his trip, all he wanted for graduation was a new car. When he
returned, his heart had changed. He asked himself, "Do I really need a new car?"
He had just left children who didn't have the basic necessities of life, like running

water, food, shelter, or an education. He thought to himself, "I have a lot of stuff and resources galore." He wanted a car, but the children he had worked with would have been happy with just a bottle of water. Because of his experience, his perspective on life had changed. He decided he wanted to start a nonprofit to serve children. He explained to me that seventy-five million children globally don't have access to education.

Taylor has volunteered at the pantry, joined a mentoring program at his school, and promised to help me lead a group of children on a trip to Ghana. I pray that God's angels protect him as he continues to use his gifts to inspire and educate children around the world. I told him he was right not to sweat not having a new car. His blessings would be hundredfold!

Be Positive

Instill the virtues of a healthy lifestyle while kids are young so they carry these values into adulthood.

Be Fruitful

BREAKFAST: Southwestern Omelet

Whisk ¾ cup liquid egg substitute with ¼ teaspoon chili powder. Heat a nonstick skillet with ½ teaspoon extra-virgin olive oil on medium-high heat and sauté ½ cup chopped onions and ¼ cup chopped red bell pepper for 2 to 3 minutes. Lower heat to medium; pour in eggs and cook until set.

Fold omelet in half and top with 2 tablespoons salsa. Warm 1 small whole-wheat tortilla (about 70 calories), if desired. Serve on the side. Complete meal with 1 small tangerine. Enjoy breakfast with a cup of coffee or tea, or another calorie-free beverage.

> 390 calories, 28 grams protein, 43 grams carbohydrate,
> 14 grams fat, 6 grams fiber

SNACK: Roast Beef and Cheddar on Crackers

Divide equally ½ ounce low-fat, low-sodium, deli-style roast beef and ½ ounce low-fat sharp cheddar cheese on 3 reduced-fat whole-wheat crackers. Enjoy with an 8-ounce glass of water.

> 100 calories, 8 grams protein, 10 grams carbohydrate,
> 3 grams fat, 2 grams fiber

LUNCH: Coconut Dream Shake

Combine 1 packet of Chocolate Shakeology mix (or 6 ounces of any low-sugar protein powder), 1 teaspoon coconut extract, ½ cup fat-free milk, 1 cup water, and ice to taste (add more ice for a thicker shake). Mix in blender until creamy.

> 200 calories, 21 grams protein, 28 grams carbohydrate,
> 1 gram fat, 3 grams fiber

SNACK: Soy Nuts and Raisins

Enjoy 1½ tablespoons dry-roasted, unsalted soy beans and 2 teaspoons raisins.

> 100 calories, 6 grams protein, 11 grams carbohydrate,
> 4 grams fat, 3 grams fiber

DINNER: Chicken in Creamy Mushroom Sauce

Cut 6 ounces boneless, skinless chicken breast into 1-inch pieces; season with ⅛ teaspoon black pepper. Set aside. Melt 1½ tablespoons low-fat buttery spread in a medium skillet. Brown chicken on both sides, about 5 minutes, adding up to 2 tablespoons fat-free, low-sodium chicken broth, if necessary, to prevent sticking. Add ¼ cup mushrooms, ⅓ cup fat-free, low-sodium chicken broth, and 1 teaspoon lemon juice. Bring to a boil, then reduce heat to a simmer. Cover and cook 15 to 20 minutes or until chicken is done. Add 1 tablespoon chopped green onions and 2 tablespoons low-fat sour cream to the chicken mixture. Cook a few minutes more until hot.

Tossed Vegetable Salad

Toss 1½ cups chopped romaine lettuce with ⅓ cup sliced green bell peppers, ⅓ cup chopped cucumber, and ¼ cup alfalfa sprouts. Drizzle with ½ teaspoon extra-virgin olive oil, 1 tablespoon balsamic vinegar, and ⅛ teaspoon black pepper.

Garlic Roast Potatoes

Preheat oven to 400°F. Coat a baking sheet with cooking spray. Toss ¾ cup diced potatoes with ⅓ cup chopped onions, 1 teaspoon chopped garlic, and 1 teaspoon extra-virgin olive oil. Season to taste with salt and pepper. Place on baking sheet in single layer. Bake for 30 to 45 minutes or until potatoes are golden and tender.

Dessert: Strawberries

Enjoy 15 whole fresh strawberries dipped in 2 tablespoons fat-free whipped topping.

> 610 calories, 44 grams protein, 60 grams carbohydrate,
> 6 grams fat, 11 grams fiber

Be Joyful

SONG OF THE DAY: "Steal Away" by Robbie Dupree

Be Fit

WARM-UP: 3–5 minutes

CARDIO: 30–60 minutes

STRENGTH TRAINING: Donnamite Ballet

STRETCH: 3–5 minutes

The Donnamite Ballet Workout

Tendu and Plié

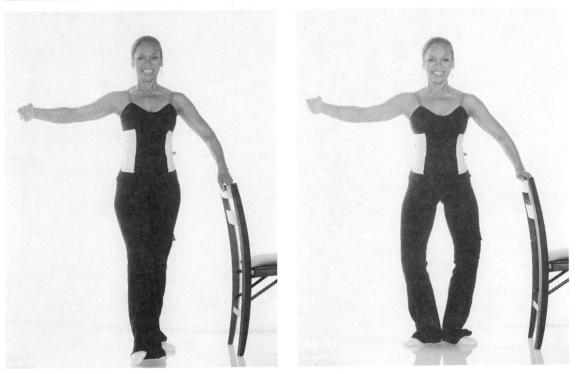

Position A   **Position B**

Stand tall with your feet in first position: the balls of the feet are turned out completely, the heels touch each other, and the feet turn outward as close as possible to a straight line. Rest one arm on top of a chair back and extend the other arm out to the side at shoulder level. Contract your abs, lift your chest, and push your shoulders and tailbone down. Slide one foot forward with your heel lifted and your toes pointed (Position A), then slide your foot back to the starting position. This is a tendu. Bend your knees over your toes (Position B), then straighten your legs again by tightening your inner thighs. This is a plié. Repeat the tendu 4 times each to the front, to the side, to the back, and to the side again, with a plié following each tendu direction. Switch legs and repeat.

Dégagé and Relevé

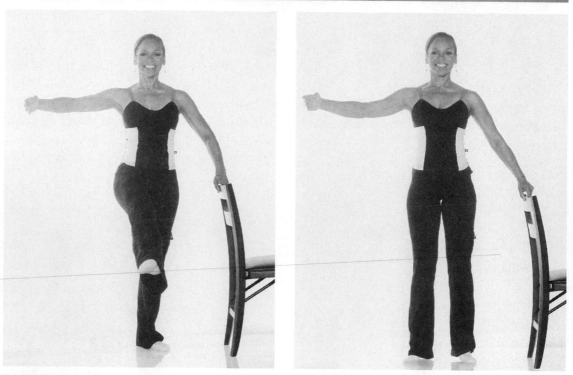

Position A   **Position B**

Start in first position as above. Brush your foot and lift it forward off the floor (Position A), then return your foot to first position. This is a dégagé. Repeat the movement to the side, to the back, and to the side, then return your foot to the starting position. Come up onto the balls of your feet, lifting your heels off the floor while keeping your legs straight (Position B), then lower yourself back down. This is a relevé. Do 4 sets each on the right and left sides.

Plié and Jump

Stand tall, facing the chair, with your hands resting on top of the back and your feet in first position. Bend your knees (Position A) and jump, landing with bended knees (Position B), then straighten your legs. Perform 8 times. Perform a tendu (slide one foot forward with heel lifted and toes pointed, then slide your foot back to the starting position). Move into second position, which is similar to first position but with feet spread apart. Bend your knees, jump, and land with bended knees, then straighten your legs. Do this 8 times. (Be sure to keep your tailbone down).

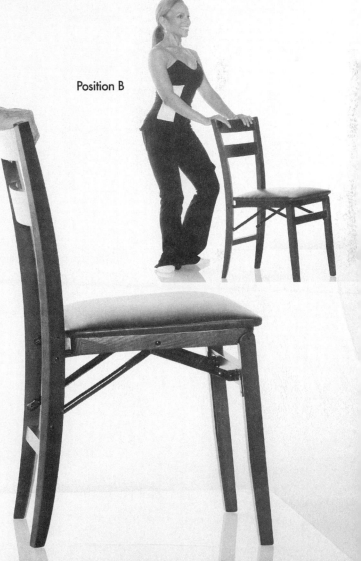

Position B

Position A

Échappé

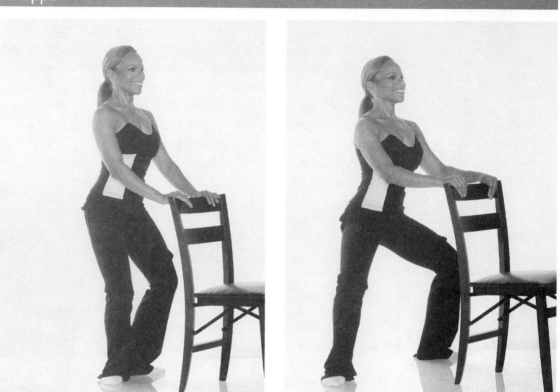

Position A   **Position B**

Start by facing a chair. Stand with your feet together in first position and bend your knees in a plié (Position A). Jump out to land in second position in a plié (Position B). Jump again, bringing your legs back together to land in first position in a plié. (This is a modified échappé.) Do 8 times.

REPEAT CIRCUIT 1–3 TIMES.

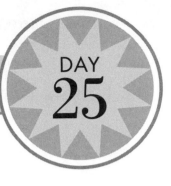
Be Faithful

*My brothers, count it all joy when you fall into diverse
temptations; Knowing this, that the trying of your faith
works patience. But let patience have her perfect work, that
you may be perfect and entire, wanting nothing.*

—JAMES 1:2–4

Be Grateful

ANNA'S STORY

*Every morning on her way to work, Anna listened to the Tom Joyner Morning
Show. The radio show was a morning treat that uplifted her spirits. At the time,
she was raising her daughter, working full-time, going to school, and trying
to make ends meet. She had run out of money, but her goal was to finish her
undergraduate studies, then to obtain her master's degree and teach children.
Every Wednesday, Tom grants a listener a "Christmas wish." On this day he read
Anna's letter and granted her the funds to continue in school.*

*She faced some financial problems after that, but she never gave up on herself.
Thank God for her family and friends, who helped support her during her ten-
year journey. They pitched in to help her and her daughter, and at last it was
time for her daughter to attend college. Anna was thrilled because she and her
daughter would attend school together. Her daughter was an undergraduate, and
Anna was in graduate school. The new goal was for them to graduate together,
but her daughter got pregnant during her last semester of school. Despite this,
Anna went on to graduate. "To God be the glory." Upon receiving her diploma,
Anna was given a Spirit Award because she motivated and empowered others.*

*She received her degree in early childhood education and went on to teach
children at schools and churches. After serving as the director of a child care
center, she enthusiastically accepted a position as the director of a YMCA. The
first program she was asked to implement was Grow Green Get Fit, which focused
on teaching kids to be healthy physically, nutritionally, and environmentally. She*

got goose bumps when she read in the manual that the program was created and written by me, Donna Richardson Joyner! She said to herself, "Look at how God works. Good humanity still exists!" After successfully completing the program, she was scheduled to speak at the National Black Child Development Institute conference with me but could not afford to attend. Before I spoke on the panel, the institute's director told me Anna's story, and I said, "Look at God." Anna is now teaching Grow Green Get Fit again, and she believes she is right on track to do her life's work. She shared with me a vision of having her own child care center, and when she does we will say again, "God is good!"

Be Positive

Keep looking up, and stop looking down.
Saddle up and stand your ground!

Be Fruitful

BREAKFAST: Hot Pumpkin Breakfast Pudding

Whisk together ¼ cup liquid egg substitute, 2 tablespoons water, 1 ounce low-fat cream cheese, and ⅓ cup fat-free ricotta cheese. Mix in ½ can pumpkin puree and ⅛ teaspoon pumpkin pie spice.

Heat in a saucepan over medium-low heat for about 5 minutes, whisking often. Add 2 tablespoons ground flax seeds and whisk well. Continue to cook for another minute. Transfer to a serving bowl and top with ¼ teaspoon unsalted butter and 1 tablespoon reduced-calorie pancake syrup. If desired, sprinkle with a bit more pumpkin pie spice or cinnamon. Serve with an 8-ounce glass of fat-free milk. Or you can pour some of the milk over the breakfast pudding and drink the rest.

> 420 calories, 29 grams protein, 43 grams carbohydrate,
> 4.5 grams fat, 8 grams fiber

SNACK: Crunchy Ham, Cheese, and Veggie Stacks

Spread 1 teaspoon low-fat mayonnaise on 1 low-sodium rye crispbread cracker. Arrange ⅓ sliced carrot and ¼ sliced cucumber on the crispbread cracker; top with ½ ounce lean, reduced-sodium ham and 1 slice low-fat Swiss cheese. Sprinkle with sodium-free spices and herbs of choice, such as freshly ground black pepper. Enjoy with a calorie-free beverage.

> 120 calories, 9 grams protein, 12 grams carbohydrate,
> 3.5 grams fat, 3 grams fiber

LUNCH: Apple in the Tropics Shake

Combine 1 packet of Tropical Strawberry Shakeology mix (or 6 ounces of any low-sugar protein powder), 1 cup unsweetened almond milk, ¼ cup unsweetened applesauce, and ice to taste (add more ice for a thicker shake). Blend until creamy.

> 226 calories, 16 grams protein, 29 grams carbohydrate,
> 4 grams fat, 3 grams fiber

SNACK: Edamame

Crunch on ½ cup steamed or boiled edamame for this easy snack. Serve with an 8-ounce glass of water.

> 100 calories, 8 grams protein, 9 grams carbohydrate,
> 3 grams fat, 4 grams fiber

DINNER: Spiced Cod

Preheat oven to 425°F. Line a baking sheet with aluminum foil. Place 6½ ounces of codfish on the prepared baking sheet. In a small bowl, combine ¼ teaspoon ground cumin, ⅛ teaspoon ground ginger, ⅛ teaspoon salt, and ⅛ teaspoon paprika. Stir in 1 tablespoon extra-virgin olive oil. Brush both sides of fish with seasoned oil. Bake fish for 10 to 15 minutes, or until fish flakes easily with a fork.

Green Bean Amandine

Steam 1 cup fresh green beans in the microwave or on the stove until crisp-tender; drain. While still warm, toss with ¼ teaspoon extra-virgin olive oil and ½ teaspoon slivered almonds.

Black Beans and Rice

Coat a small skillet with cooking spray. Heat on medium. Add ¾ teaspoon chopped onion and sauté for 3 to 4 minutes until translucent. Place 2 table-spoons cooked black beans in a small saucepan. Mix in onions, 1 teaspoon fresh chopped cilantro, 1 teaspoon chopped garlic, ⅛ teaspoon ground cumin, and ⅛ teaspoon black pepper. Throw in one bay leaf. Bring to a boil. Reduce heat and simmer for 10 to 15 minutes. Remove bay leaf. Pour hot beans over 5 tablespoons cooked white rice.

Raspberry Gelatin Dessert

Prepare your favorite flavor of dry-mix gelatin per package directions. Portion out ½ cup and top with 2 tablespoons raspberries and 1 tablespoon fat-free whipped topping.

> 590 calories, 44 grams protein, 54 grams carbohydrate,
> 21 grams fat, 8 grams fiber

Be Joyful

SONG OF THE DAY: "Peg" by Steely Dan

Be Fit

WARM-UP: 3–4 minutes
CARDIO: 30–60 minutes
STRENGTH TRAINING: Strong and Sexy
STRETCH: 3–5 minutes

Strong and Sexy Workout

Balance Lunge

Stand with your feet shoulder-width apart, letting your arms hang at your sides. Bend your right knee and lift it to hip level while you raise your arms overhead with palms together (Position A). Hold for 3–5 seconds, then lower your right foot into a front lunge, keeping your arms above your head (Position B). Push off your right foot and return to the starting position. Repeat on the left side. Perform 12–15 reps.

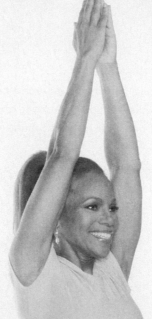

Position A

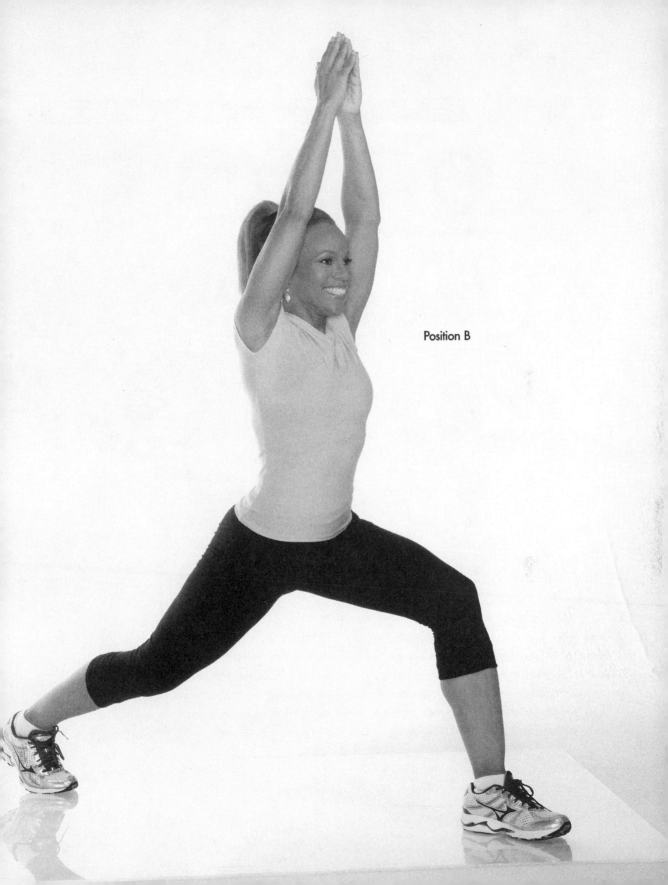

Position B

Bicep Balance

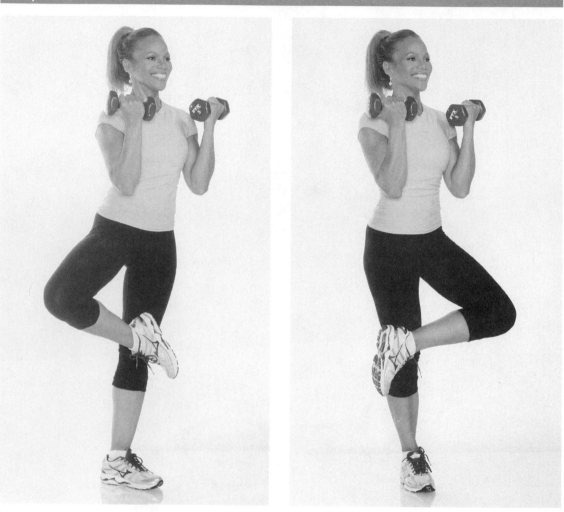

Position A   **Position B**

Stand tall with weights in your hands and lift your right foot across the left thigh, letting your arms hang at your sides. Your right knee will be pointed to the side, and your abs should be contracted. Balance and lift the weights toward your shoulders (Position A), then lower the weights back to the starting position. Switch sides and lift the left foot across the right thigh, letting your arms hang down, then slowly balance and lift the weights toward your shoulders (Position B). Perform 12–15 reps on each side.

Calf Raise and Tricep Kickback

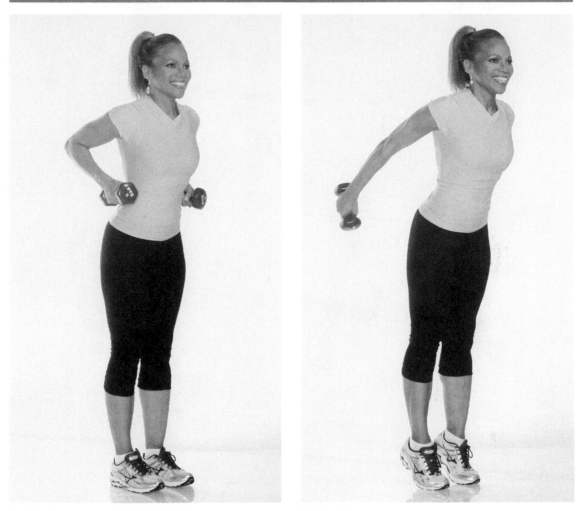

Position A   **Position B**

Stand tall with a slight forward lean, your feet hip-width apart, your arms bent with elbows pointing back, and weights in your hands (Position A). Roll up onto the balls of your feet and extend your arms back (Position B). Lower your heels to the floor, bending your arms and bringing the weights back to your sides. Perform 12–15 reps.

Lunge and Deltoid Raise

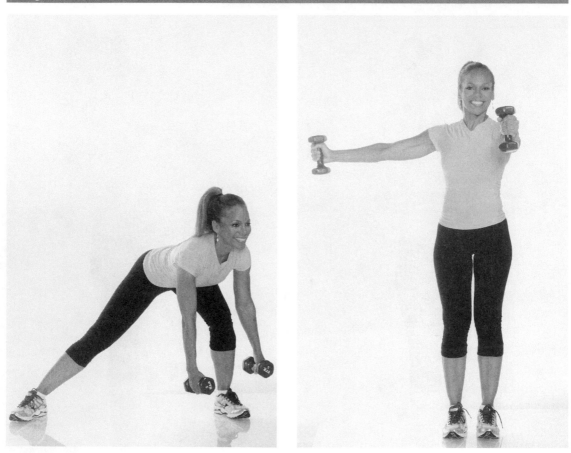

Position A   Position B

Stand tall with your feet hip-width apart and your arms at your sides with weights in your hands. Step into a left side lunge and lower the weights to your left foot (Position A). Push off the left foot and return to the starting position. Lift your left arm forward to shoulder height and your right arm out to the side at shoulder height (Position B). Return to the starting position with your arms by your sides. Repeat on the other side. Perform 12–15 reps.

REPEAT CIRCUIT 1–3 TIMES.

Be Faithful

*That every one of you should know how to possess
his vessel in sanctification and honor.*
—1 THESSALONIANS 4:4

Be Grateful

WANDA'S STORY

I have heard the horror stories. I have witnessed those flashes of heat and the sudden removal of clothing. I have seen the abrupt changes in mood and behavior in family, friends, and colleagues. However, my assistant Wanda is one of the few people I have ever talked to about menopause who has a truly positive attitude about it. Despite every negative comment or stereotype—such as the night sweats, depression, irritability, weight gain, and dry skin—Wanda has turned those negatives around and approaches them with a positive outlook.

Wanda said that she first had to think about this new phase in her life with a positive and proactive attitude. She eats healthier now and includes vitamins and minerals in her daily routine. She says her homeopathic choices have helped her so much that she forgets she is even in menopause. Wanda includes more organic foods and lots of fruits and vegetables. She said some of her Caribbean friends told her to add a little flaxseed to her meals to reduce her hot flashes. As far as she is concerned, they were spot-on; she has yet to strip down in public because of those flashes. She also uses lots of aloe vera—both internally and externally. She takes a full aloe leaf, blends it with water, and drinks the juice a couple of times a month to aid with digestive issues faced during menopause, and she uses the plant externally for dry skin and as a remedy for other skin ailments.

There is an abundance of information at your local health food store, at the nearest farmers' market, and at your local library that can make the transition into this stage of your life fun, exciting, and healthy. Stay positive like Wanda, and enjoy every moment of being a woman!

Be Positive

Declare a new season for yourself by embracing healthy living and well-being. You can't change your past health, but you can change your future health.

Be Fruitful

BREAKFAST: Strawberry-Ricotta Breakfast Wrap

Arrange ⅓ cup fresh sliced strawberries down the center of a 6-inch low-carb whole-wheat tortilla. Spoon ⅔ cup fat-free ricotta cheese over the strawberries. Roll tortilla up, place seam-side down on a microwave-safe plate, and cover loosely with plastic wrap. Microwave on high for about 1 minute, or until ricotta cheese is heated through. Sprinkle with 2 tablespoons chopped walnuts. Serve immediately with a 6-ounce glass of fat-free milk.

> 390 calories, 27 grams protein, 40 grams carbohydrate,
> 12 grams fat, 10 grams fiber

SNACK: Roast Beef and Cheddar on Crackers

Divide equally ½ ounce low-fat, low-sodium, deli-style roast beef and ½ ounce low-fat sharp cheddar cheese on 3 reduced-fat whole-wheat crackers. Enjoy with an 8-ounce glass of water.

> 100 calories, 8 grams protein, 10 grams carbohydrate,
> 3 grams fat, 2 grams fiber

LUNCH: Tea-Berry Zinger Shake

Combine 1 packet of Greenberry Shakeology mix (or 6 ounces of any low-sugar protein powder), 1 cup cold unsweetened green tea, 1 cup raspberries, and ice to taste (add more ice for a thicker shake). Blend until creamy.

> 205 calories, 16 grams protein, 35 grams carbohydrate,
> 1.5 grams fat, 3 grams fiber

SNACK: Seafood Salad with Celery Stalks

Shred 2 ounces imitation crab and mix with 1½ teaspoons low-fat mayonnaise and ⅛ teaspoon dried dill weed. Serve with 3 celery stalks. Enjoy with an 8-ounce glass of water.

> 110 calories, 9 grams protein, 11 grams carbohydrate,
> 3 grams fat, 2 grams fiber

DINNER: Herb-Roasted Chicken and Vegetables

Preheat oven to 450°F. Rinse 6 ounces boneless, skinless chicken breast, remove any visible fat, and pat dry with a paper towel. Place in the middle of a baking pan lightly coated with nonstick cooking spray. Wash and peel ⅓ eggplant with a vegetable peeler and cut into 1-inch pieces. Place the eggplant, ¼ cup onion, and 1 teaspoon chopped garlic in a large bowl. Drizzle with 2½ teaspoons extra-virgin olive oil and stir lightly to combine. Spread the vegetables around the chicken.

Chop ½ medium tomato coarsely; place on top of the vegetables. Sprinkle chicken with ⅛ teaspoon dried basil, ⅛ teaspoon dried oregano, ⅛ teaspoon salt, and ⅛ teaspoon black pepper, or to taste. Roast in the oven for 10 minutes. Turn the chicken and gently stir the vegetable mixture. Return to oven and roast for an additional 10 to 15 minutes, or until chicken is no longer pink inside and vegetables are tender.

Garlic Roast Potatoes

Preheat oven to 400°F. Coat a baking sheet with cooking spray. Toss together ¾ cup diced potatoes, ⅓ cup chopped onions, 1 teaspoon chopped garlic, and 1 teaspoon extra-virgin olive oil. Season to taste with salt and pepper. Place on baking sheet in single layer. Bake potatoes for approximately 30 to 45 minutes or until potatoes are golden and tender.

Dessert: Honeydew and Grapes

Enjoy ¾ cup honeydew melon balls and ⅓ cup grapes (any color) for dessert.

> 590 calories, 41 grams protein, 63 grams carbohydrate,
> 21 grams fat, 12 grams fiber

Be Joyful

SONG OF THE DAY: "SexyBack" by Justin Timberlake

Be Fit

WARM-UP: 3–5 minutes
CARDIO: 30–60 minutes
STRENGTH TRAINING: High School Reunion
STRETCH: 3–5 minutes

High School Reunion Workout

Bicycle

Lie on your back with your right leg bent at a 90-degree angle and your hands behind your head. Contract your abs, lift your head off the floor, and rotate your torso so that your left shoulder points toward your right knee (Position A). Cycle your legs, raising your left leg and straightening your right while lifting your right shoulder to point toward your left knee (Position B). Continue to cycle your legs, alternately lifting your shoulders. Perform 15 reps.

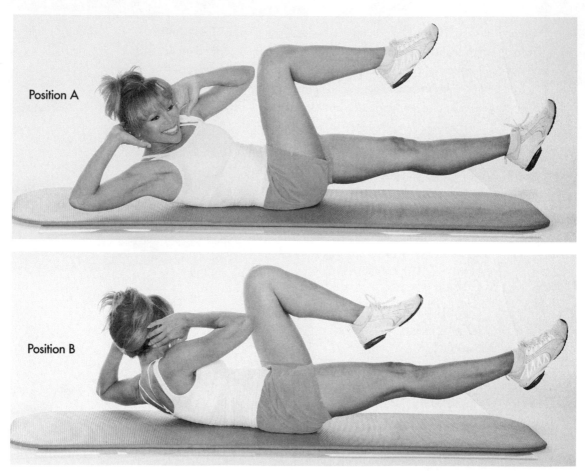

Position A

Position B

Side Plank Reach-Through

Start in a plank position supported by your forearms and toes (Position A). Rotate your body to a side plank position, then reach your arm across your chest toward your back (Position B). Bring your arm back in and return to a side plank. Return to the starting position. Repeat the exercise series. Perform 15 reps and repeat on the other side.

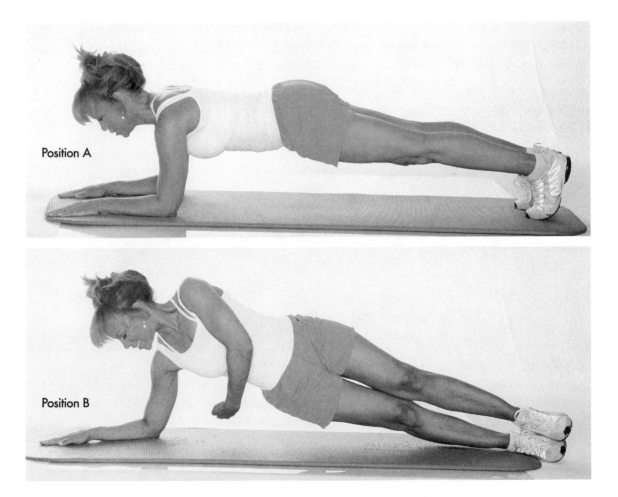

Position A

Position B

Push-Up

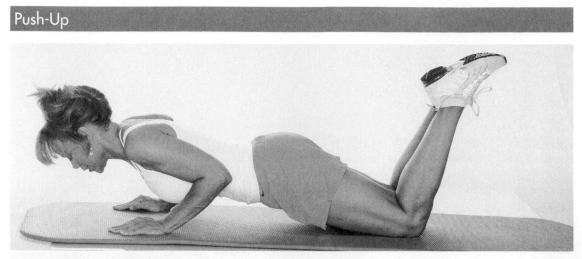

Exercise 3

Start on your hands and knees with your legs bent and your feet in the air. Your arms should be straight with your hands shoulder-width apart. Bend your arms with your elbows pointing back as you lower your chest to the floor. Push into the palms of your hands to lift up to the starting position. Perform 15 reps.

Hip Abduction

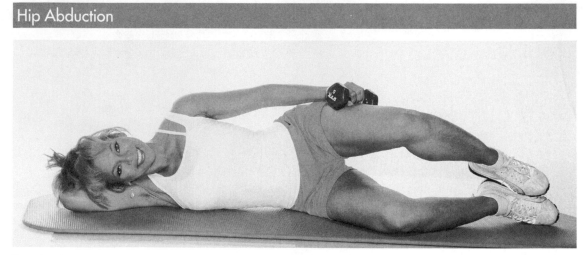

Exercise 4

Lie on your right side, with your head resting on your right arm, your hips stacked, your feet together, and your legs slightly bent. Hold a weight in your left hand, resting it on your left thigh. Lift up your left thigh, then lower it to the start position. Perform 15 reps, then switch sides and repeat.

Swan

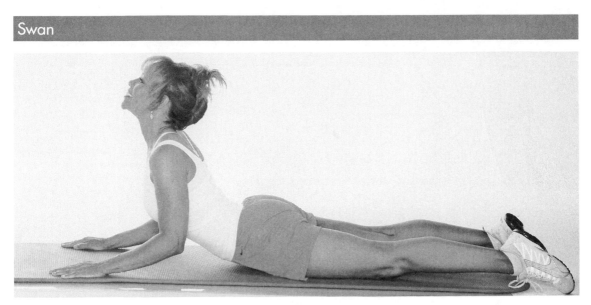

Exercise 5

Lie facedown with your arms bent, your hands under your shoulders, your legs extended, and your feet together. Contract your buttocks, tighten your abs, and draw your shoulders down and back. Inhale and lift your chest off the mat. Exhale, hold, then lower. Do 5 sets.

Swimming

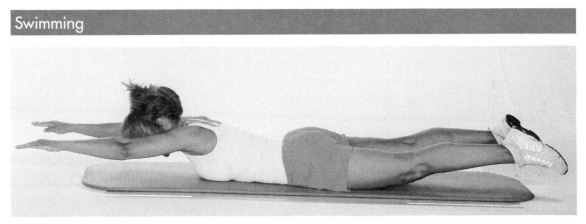

Exercise 6

Lie facedown, your arms extended above your head and your legs straight, with your shoulders down and back. Inhale and lift the arms, chest, and legs, tightening the abs. Flutter your arms and legs simultaneously. Hold for 8 counts, then lower. Do 5 sets.

REPEAT CIRCUIT 1–3 TIMES.

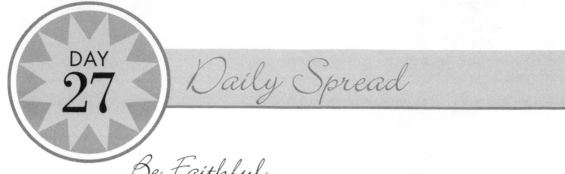

Be Faithful

*He gives power to the faint; and to them that
have no might he increases strength.*

—ISAIAH 40:29

Be Grateful

MONTY'S STORY

*I was at a family gathering when my friend said to me, "Look around. What do
you see?" I told him, "I see my family, love, and community." Then he said, "If
you look carefully, you see obesity." He was right. I have never really paid much
attention to the health of my family. Since then I have asked myself why we in
the United States are obsessed with processed foods, reluctant to move our bodies,
and resistant to taking accountability for our own health? Is it that we don't care
enough to do something about it? I decided to do something about my health and
become a role model. "To whom much is given, much is required." God puts you
in a place, then he expects a lot from you.*

*My body needed to exemplify my trust in him so I could be a greater witness.
God will take away what he has given us if we don't use it. This is especially true
in regard to our health and well-being. I had to take control of my health and
not get caught up in what I didn't like about my body; instead I needed to focus
on improving myself. Change was necessary for me to lose weight and keep the
weight off. My whole being was affected by my weight loss—my marriage, my job,
and my spiritual life. I had to have the right attitude, willpower, and willingness
to change.*

*Once my mind-set changed, I had the ability to do new and different things.
I became a better person, and I was able to help other people. I wanted to be a
better husband and father. My wife was happy to see me get up at 5:15 A.M. to go
work out. She saw me doing something positive. She was inspired, and now she is
helping people by giving free massages to breast cancer survivors. Our relationship*

is stronger, and now my wife and I love salsa dancing. In the past, I would not have been open to trying it, but I have learned to think and do things differently. The change also affected my work. My goal is now to help my colleagues become open to new possibilities. I arrive at work fresh, open to new thinking, and ready to accomplish things beyond my previous expectations. I'm no longer limited in my thinking, and I have the courage to continue to change.

Monty

Be Positive

Do not call to mind former things or ponder events of the past. Focus your energies on reaching.

Be Fruitful

BREAKFAST: Chocolate Spice Shake

Combine 1 packet of Chocolate Shakeology mix (or 6 ounces of any low-sugar protein powder), 1 teaspoon cinnamon, ½ teaspoon nutmeg, 1 cup fat-free milk, and ice to taste (add more ice for a thicker shake). Blend until creamy.

232 calories, 25 grams protein, 32 grams carbohydrate, 1 gram fat, 3 grams fiber

SNACK: Pesto-Artichoke Chicken Wrap

Shred 2 tablespoons cooked chicken. In a small bowl, combine shredded chicken, 2½ teaspoons coarsely chopped artichoke hearts (fresh, cooked, or canned), and ½ teaspoon fresh chopped scallions. Set aside. Spread ½ teaspoon pesto sauce on a 6-inch low-carb flour tortilla. Arrange chicken mix and 1 piece of pimento on top. Roll up tortilla; heat if desired. Enjoy with an 8-ounce glass of water.

120 calories, 9 grams protein, 13 grams carbohydrate, 3.5 grams fat, 8 grams fiber

LUNCH: Tuna and Tomato Salad

Mix 3 ounces tuna (canned in water, drained), 5 halved cherry tomatoes, 3 jumbo olives, 2 teaspoons extra-virgin olive oil, and 2 teaspoons white rice vinegar in a bowl; mix lightly. Place on bed of lettuce (2 cups chopped romaine). Serve with ¾ cup grapes (any color) and a calorie-free beverage.

320 calories, 24 grams protein, 31 carbohydrate, 12 grams fat, 5 grams fiber

SNACK: Edamame

Crunch on ½ cup steamed or boiled edamame for this easy snack. Serve with an 8-ounce glass of water.

100 calories, 8 grams protein, 9 grams carbohydrate, 3 grams fat, 4 grams fiber

DINNER: Grilled Steak with Salsa Sauce

Mix together 3 tablespoons salsa and 2 tablespoons reduced-fat sour cream; refrigerate until ready to serve.

Trim any fat from 6 ounces lean, ⅛-inch-trim top sirloin. Season with ⅛ teaspoon black pepper and ⅛ teaspoon garlic powder. Grill the steak 4 to 5 minutes on each side, turning once, for medium-rare, or longer to desired doneness. Transfer the steak to a cutting board and let rest for 5 minutes; slice on the diagonal into ½-inch-thick slices. To serve, spoon the salsa mixture onto a plate and place the steak slices, slightly overlapping, on top.

Spinach Salad

Halve 4 cherry tomatoes and toss with 1¼ cup fresh, chopped spinach and ¼ cup sliced mushrooms. Drizzle with 1½ teaspoons reduced-fat ranch dressing and 1 tablespoon balsamic vinegar.

Cottage Fries

Prepare 12 cottage-cut frozen french fries per package directions. Serve with 1 tablespoon ketchup.

Dessert: Grilled Ginger Pineapple

Top 4 pieces sliced pineapple (canned in water) with equally divided 1½ teaspoons packed brown sugar and ½ teaspoon fresh chopped ginger. Place under broiler and cook until sugar begins to caramelize.

560 calories, 45 grams protein, 59 grams carbohydrate, 7 grams fat, 6 grams fiber

Be Joyful

SONG OF THE DAY: "(I Can't Get No) Satisfaction" by the Rolling Stones

Be Fit

WARM-UP: 3–5 minutes
CARDIO: 30–60 minutes
STRENGTH TRAINING: Champions
STRETCH: 3–5 minutes

Champions
Workout

Golf Move

Exercise 1

Stand in an athletic position and bend at the hips, your knees over your heels, and your hands together in front of you as if holding a golf club. Rotate your torso and swing your arms back, then rotate your torso back around and swing through as if you were taking a golf swing. Return to the start position. Perform 10 swings, then jog in place for 10 counts. Repeat on the same side for 2 minutes. Perform this exercise on the right if you are right-handed or on the left if you are left-handed.

Exercise 2

Stand tall. Jump with your right foot forward and your left foot back while extending your left arm forward and your right arm back. Then jump again, switching to the left foot forward and the right foot back, while extending your right arm forward and your left arm back. Perform for 2 minutes.

Volleyball Move

Exercise 3

Start in a squat position with your arms hanging down and your hands clasped together. Straighten your legs and at the same time lift your hands as if you were hitting a volleyball. Perform 10 volleys, then jump up with your arms overhead as if you were hitting the ball over the edge of the net for 10 reps. Alternate movements for 2 minutes.

Basketball Move

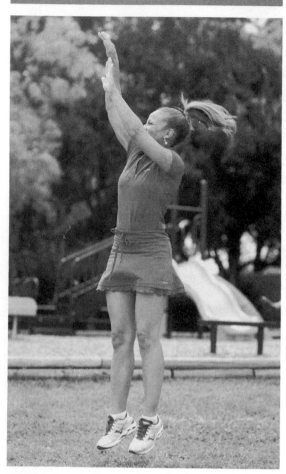

Football Move

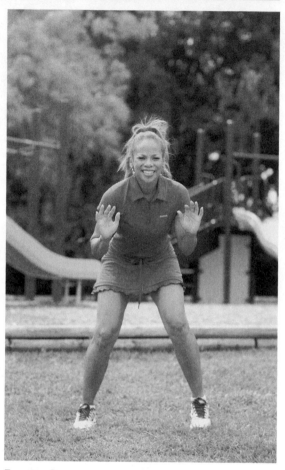

Exercise 4

Pretend you are dribbling a basketball to the right with your right hand for 6 counts, then shoot on counts 7 and 8. Repeat on the left. Alternate sides and perform for 2 minutes.

Exercise 5

Start in an athletic squat position on the balls of your feet. Run in place for a few steps, then turn ¼ turn to the right and continue to run in place. Turn another ¼ turn to the right and continue to run in place. Perform for 2 minutes, circling around a few times.

Boxing Move

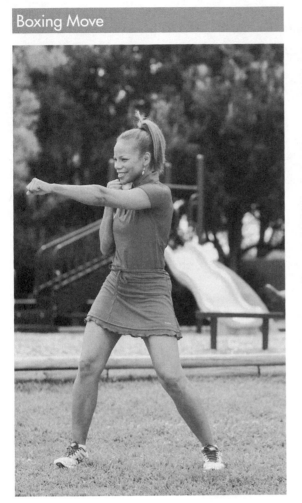

Tennis Move

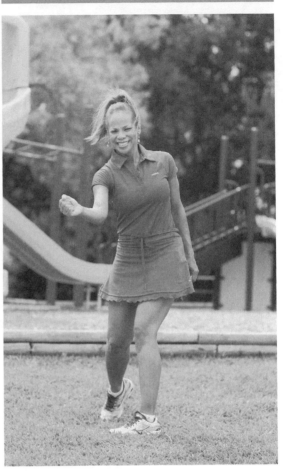

Exercise 6

Stand tall and shuffle your feet to the right for 3 counts, then with a clenched fist extend your left hand in a quick jab motion across your chest to the right. Shuffle your feet to the left for 3 counts, then with a clenched fist extend your right hand across your chest to the left. Perform exercise for 2 minutes, alternating sides.

Exercise 7

Jog to the right for 6 counts, then step, pivot, and swing through as though you were using a tennis racket to hit a ball. Jog to the left for 6 counts, then step, pivot, and swing through as though holding a tennis racket to hit a ball. Alternate sides and perform for 2 minutes.

Soccer Move

Exercise 8

Start in an athletic squat position with your arms bent at your sides. Stepping forward with your left foot, kick out with your right foot. Jog in place for 3 counts, then return to the starting position. Repeat exercise. Perform for 1 minute. Switch to the other leg, and perform exercise for 1 minute.

**REPEAT CIRCUIT
1–3 TIMES.**

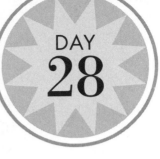
Be Faithful

Do not grieve, for the joy of the
Lord is your strength.
—NEHEMIAH 8:10

Be Grateful

BONNIE'S STORY

Everyone in the health and fitness industry knows who Bonnie Prudden is. In the 1940s and 1950s, Bonnie was known as a dancer and a rock climber. She was distinguished in over thirty documented first ascents and as a conditioning instructor. Back in the day, Bonnie used to tell her students, "You can't turn back the clock, but you can wind it up again." Spoken like a true no-nonsense woman who decided after watching her daughter's gym classes in the 1940s to use her background in dance and athletics to give conditioning classes for the neighborhood children.

As the classes grew, she tested the students' progress in muscular fitness and noticed that new students failed the test but returning students passed. Bonnie went on to test thousands of children across America and Europe and found that Americans were the least fit. The results were presented to President Dwight Eisenhower at a White House luncheon in 1955 in what is known as the "report that shocked the president" and led Eisenhower to establish the President's Council on Youth Fitness.

In November 2007, the President's Council on Physical Fitness and Sports awarded Bonnie, then age ninety-three, the inaugural Lifetime Achievement Award. She was chosen based on the span and scope of her career, the number of lives she had touched through her work, the legacy of her work, and additional honors she had received during her career.

Thanks to fitness pioneer Bonnie Prudden, I have had the honor to serve on the President's Council on Fitness, Sports, and Nutrition under President George Bush and President Barack Obama.

I serve with humility and grace and will continue to help America live an abundantly healthy life.

Be Positive

Shake off your past mistakes. Focus on what is in front of you, not what is behind you. Don't let anything stop your mission.

Be Fruitful

BREAKFAST: Raspberries and Walnuts

Pour ¾ cup whole-grain cereal into a bowl and add 1 cup fat-free milk, 1½ tablespoons chopped walnuts, and ⅓ cup raspberries. Enjoy with a piece of low-fat string cheese on the side. Serve with a cup of coffee or tea, lightened with ½ cup (4 ounces) fat-free milk.

420 calories, 28 grams protein, 50 grams carbohydrate,
4.5 grams fat, 8 grams fiber

SNACK: Cottage Cheese and Strawberries

Top ⅓ cup low-fat (1%) cottage cheese with 6 whole fresh strawberries and 1½ teaspoons chopped pecans. Enjoy with an 8-ounce glass of water.

110 calories, 9 grams protein, 13 grams carbohydrate,
4 grams fat, 2 grams fiber

LUNCH: Coconut Twist Shake

Combine 1 packet of Tropical Strawberry Shakeology mix (or 6 ounces of any low-sugar protein powder), 1 cup coconut water, 2 tablespoons 100% grapefruit juice, ½ cup unsweetened pineapple chunks, and ice to taste (add more ice for a thicker shake). Blend until creamy.

259 calories, 17.5 grams protein, 42.5 grams carbohydrate,
1.5 grams fat, 3 grams fiber

SNACK: Ham-Wrapped Dates

Cut 1½ ounces thinly sliced low-sodium ham into 2 strips. Wrap ham strips around 2 whole dates and enjoy with a glass of water.

120 calories, 10 grams protein, 13 grams carbohydrate,
3.5 grams fat, 1 gram fiber

DINNER: Parmesan-Dijon Chicken

Preheat oven to 375°F. Mix 1½ tablespoons seasoned bread crumbs with
1 tablespoon fat-free Parmesan cheese and spread out on a plate. Melt
1 teaspoon of low-fat buttery spread and combine with ½ teaspoon Dijon
mustard in a shallow dish. Dip chicken into spread mixture, then coat with
bread crumb mixture. Place in baking dish. Dot with 1⅓ tablespoons low-fat
buttery spread. Bake uncovered for 20 to 25 minutes, turning once, or until
chicken is no longer pink inside.

Peas and Carrots

Heat ½ cup frozen peas and carrots in a small saucepan or in the microwave
per package directions. Top with ¾ teaspoon low-fat buttery spread.

Garlic Bread

Combine 1 teaspoon low-fat buttery spread and ¼ teaspoon chopped garlic
in a small saucepan. Stir until melted. Brush mix onto ½ medium whole-wheat
hoagie roll. Sprinkle with ¼ teaspoon dried parsley. Place on baking sheet and
broil until golden.

Dessert: Chocolate-and-Nut-Coated Banana

Coat ½ small banana with 1½ tablespoons fat-free light chocolate syrup.
Sprinkle with 1 teaspoon chopped pecans. Place in refrigerator or freezer to
set. Enjoy for dessert.

600 calories, 45 grams protein, 61 grams carbohydrate,
5 grams fat, 8 grams fiber

Be Joyful

SONG OF THE DAY: "Signed, Sealed, Delivered, I'm Yours" by Stevie Wonder

Be Fit

Weekly Fitness Diary

_____

_____

_____

_____

_____

_____

_____

_____

_____

_____

_____

_____

_____

_____

_____

_____

_____

_____

_____

_____

_____

_____

_____

_____

_____

_____

Receive it! Achieve it! Believe it!

ACKNOWLEDGMENTS

I would like to acknowledge and thank the following people who helped me by nurturing my body, mind, and soul as I live out my passion and vision. In writing this book, my goal is to inspire and encourage all to receive the blessing of newness in their health.

First, thank you to God, my Lord and Savior, who makes *all things possible*! To my dad, James Richardson, and my mom, Laverne Richardson, I thank you for your unconditional love and for teaching me to love God and be true to who I am. Thanks to my family, for keeping me grounded, rooted, and focused on my purpose. Thanks to my spiritual teachers, Bishop T. D. Jakes and First Lady Serita, whose guidance has helped me to grow stronger, wiser, and spiritually whole.

Thank you to my dear friend Elder Tarra Reown, for your liquid sunshine, sweet tweets, and blessed prayers, and to my assistant, Wanda Payton, for your dedication, your hard work, and helping to keep my grooviness in check. Special thanks to my business consultant, Hattie Hill, CEO of Hattie Hill Enterprises, and the fantastic Briana Harden, and to my manager, Louis Upkins, for your love, covering, and expertise.

Thanks to the wonderful Jan Miller and Nena Madonia, my literary agents at Dupree Miller, for your belief from the very beginning in me and my message to motivate women, men, and families to make healthier choices and live more fulfilling and purposeful lives. To Michelle Adams, who captured my voice and helped me articulate and share the gospel of good health. Thank you to Nancy Hancock, Elsa Dixon, and the entire team at Harper Collins/HarperOne, for your tireless dedication to making sure we stayed on track and completed the mission. To Carl Daikeler, CEO of Beachbody, and Jeanette Corcuera, for your confidence and faith that together we could create a healthier America. Thanks to my mountaineer partner and extraordinary photographer Rance Elgin, who captures the very essence of being a witness to fitness.

Thank you to my wives prayer group—I love and treasure you all. To my sister-in-spirit Elder Cathy Moffitt, for your love and spiritual guidance. Thank you to my good friend Jacqueline Jakes, for your prayers, your support, and our "Yeah for Jesus" moments. To Coach Anna McCoy, for your wisdom, insight, and acumen for this entire book writing process.

Thank you to my countless friends, for keeping me accountable, keeping it real, and teaching me how to live in the moment.

INDEX

SCAN THIS CODE

WITH YOUR SMARTPHONE TO BE LINKED TO

THE BONUS MATERIALS FOR

WITNESS TO FITNESS

on the Elixir mobile website,
where you can also find information about other
healthy living books and related materials

YOU CAN ALSO TEXT

FITNESS to READIT (732348)

to be sent a link to the Elixir mobile website.

 Facebook.com/elixirliving   Twitter.com/elixirliving   www.elixirliving.com

Got faith? Get RESULTS.

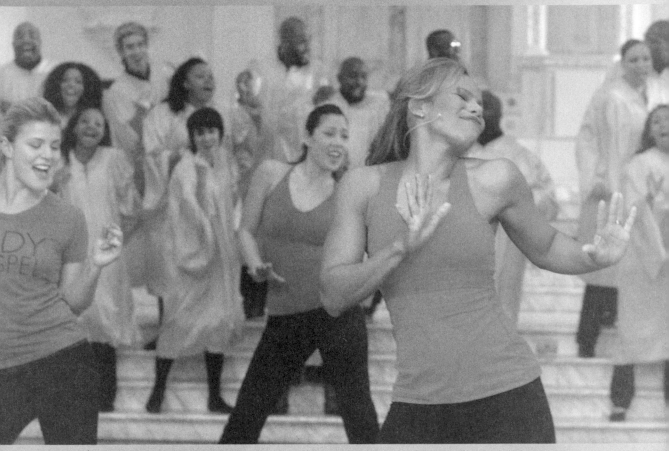

Body Gospel® is a first-of-its-kind program, including workouts set to incredible gospel music, effective resistance bands, and a complete nutrition plan created by fitness icon Donna Richardson Joyner.

Every workout is a "party with a purpose." And that purpose is to get you healthy—in mind, body, and spirit. *If you believe, you will succeed.*

Get the complete Body Gospel program—6 workouts on 3 DVDs; the Total Transformation Guide; the Feed Your Body, Feed Your Soul Nutrition Guide; the Body Gospel Training Cards; and the Body Gospel Bands, designed to engage your core and upper and lower body, all at the same time. *A $400.00 value.*

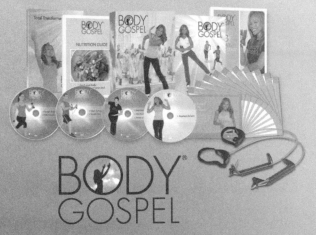

BODY®
GOSPEL